CORTISOL

The Ultimate Hormone – Enhance Your Well-being, Weight Management, Fertility, Menopause, Longevity, and Alleviate Stress

By

Calvin M. Duncan

Table Of Contents

Chapter One

Introduction

Understanding Cortisol: The Master Hormone

In the intricate web of the human endocrine system, one hormone emerges as a central orchestrator, governing a myriad of physiological processes. This sentinel of balance is cortisol, often hailed as the "master hormone" due to its pervasive influence on our health and well-being. As we delve into the complexities of cortisol, an intriguing narrative unfolds, revealing its origins, role in stress response, and far-reaching impact on various facets of our lives.

At its core, cortisol is a product of the adrenal glands, released in response to stressors as part of the body's adaptive mechanism. This fundamental nature positions cortisol as a key player in the intricate dance of the endocrine system, ensuring equilibrium in the face of challenges. The exploration of cortisol's origins takes us into the depths of the body's physiological response to stress, unveiling its adaptability and evolutionary significance.

The symbiotic relationship between cortisol and stress unveils a delicate balance. As cortisol surges during times of stress, it prompts the body to mobilize energy reserves, heighten alertness, and prepare for action. However, this finely tuned response becomes a double-edged sword when stress becomes chronic. The once adaptive cortisol surge transforms into a persistent presence, contributing to a cascade of health implications.

A profound dimension of cortisol's influence manifests in its role in weight management. The hormone exerts a nuanced impact on metabolism, fat storage, and appetite regulation. Unraveling the intricacies of this relationship provides valuable insights into the challenges many face in achieving and maintaining a healthy weight. Cortisol, in its dual role as both an ally and adversary, underscores the importance of a balanced approach to weight management.

Beyond its implications for weight, cortisol extends its influence into realms of reproductive health. The intricate connections between cortisol levels and fertility unveil a narrative of hormonal interplay. Stress, and subsequently elevated cortisol, can disrupt reproductive hormones, presenting challenges for those on the path to conception. In this context, understanding and managing cortisol levels become essential components of fertility journeys.

The menopausal transition, a transformative phase in a woman's life, also bears the imprint of cortisol's influence. As hormonal fluctuations characterize this period, cortisol adds another layer to the complexity. Exploring the role of cortisol during menopause unveils insights into the interplay of hormones, offering a holistic perspective on managing this significant life stage with grace and well-being.

The quest for longevity intertwines with the cortisol connection, shedding light on how chronic stress may impact the aging process. Cortisol's role in the body's response to stressors becomes a crucial consideration in the pursuit of a healthy and resilient life. Strategies that contribute to a balanced cortisol profile emerge as integral components of promoting longevity and well-being.

The narrative culminates in an exploration of stress and cortisol, unraveling the biochemical pathways and feedback loops that govern this intricate relationship. Chronic stress, a pervasive feature of modern life, prompts a closer examination of its consequences on overall health. Understanding the ways in which cortisol mediates the body's adaptive responses to stressors equips individuals with tools to navigate the challenges of contemporary living.

In conclusion, "Understanding Cortisol: The Master Hormone" invites readers on a journey into the inner workings of this influential hormone. From its origins to its impact on weight, fertility, menopause, and longevity, the exploration of cortisol transcends scientific inquiry, offering a compass for navigating the complexities of our health and well-being. As we grasp the significance of cortisol, we empower ourselves to foster balance and resilience in the face of life's myriad stressors.

Importance of Cortisol in Health and Well-being

In the intricate tapestry of human physiology, hormones act as messengers, orchestrating a symphony of processes essential to our well-being. Among these, cortisol emerges as a linchpin, a vital player that transcends mere biochemical function to profoundly influence our health and overall sense of well-being.

Cortisol, produced by the adrenal glands, holds the mantle of the body's primary stress hormone. Its release is intricately tied to the intricate dance of the endocrine system, responding dynamically to the ebb and flow of daily challenges. This responsiveness underscores its adaptability, positioning cortisol as a central figure in the body's coping mechanisms.

At its core, cortisol's role in the stress response is evolutionary, dating back to a time when survival often hinged on swift reactions to imminent threats. In the face of stressors, cortisol orchestrates a

cascade of physiological changes. It mobilizes energy reserves, sharpens cognitive functions, and readies the body for action. This acute stress response, often known as the "fight or flight" mechanism, is a testament to cortisol's adaptability and its crucial role in navigating challenges.

Yet, the tale of cortisol unfolds beyond acute stressors, delving into the realms of chronic stress, where its role becomes more complex. In the modern landscape, characterized by persistent stressors and a frenetic pace of life, cortisol's prolonged presence can have profound implications for health. Chronic elevation of cortisol levels is associated with a range of adverse effects, from compromised immune function to disrupted sleep patterns and metabolic imbalances.

Weight management, a cornerstone of overall health, is intricately linked to cortisol. The hormone exerts a multifaceted influence on metabolism, appetite regulation, and fat storage. While acute cortisol spikes may aid in immediate energy mobilization, chronic elevation can contribute to weight-related challenges. Understanding this delicate balance becomes essential in the context of prevailing issues such as obesity and metabolic disorders.

The impact of cortisol extends to the intricate realm of reproductive health. Fertility, a biological hallmark, can be influenced by cortisol levels. Chronic stress, and the resulting elevated cortisol, may disrupt the delicate interplay of reproductive hormones, posing challenges for those seeking to conceive. Here, the importance of managing cortisol takes on a poignant significance in the context of family planning and reproductive well-being.

As women navigate the transformative phase of menopause, cortisol adds another layer to the intricate hormonal transitions characterizing this life stage. The interplay of cortisol with other hormones during menopause underscores the need for a holistic understanding of hormonal changes. Strategies to manage cortisol levels become integral in fostering well-being during this significant period of a woman's life.

In the pursuit of longevity and resilient health, cortisol emerges as a pivotal factor. Chronic stress, often marked by sustained elevation of cortisol, is implicated in accelerated aging processes. Strategies that mitigate the impact of stress on cortisol levels become crucial in promoting not just a longer life but one marked by vitality and well-being.

In essence, the importance of cortisol in health and well-being is a narrative that traverses the realms of acute stress responses to the nuanced challenges of chronic stress in modern life. Recognizing cortisol as a central figure in this narrative empowers individuals to adopt proactive measures for stress management. From lifestyle choices to mindfulness practices, the spectrum of strategies is vast, offering a holistic approach to maintaining a balanced cortisol profile and, in turn, nurturing enduring health and well-being. As we navigate the complexities of contemporary existence, understanding and respecting the role of cortisol becomes a cornerstone of the quest for a thriving, resilient, and balanced life.

Chapter Two

Cortisol and its Role in Weight Management

In the realm of weight management, the influence of hormones is profound, and one hormone that takes center stage is cortisol. As the primary stress hormone, cortisol plays a multifaceted role in the body's response to stressors, impacting various physiological processes, including metabolism, appetite regulation, and fat storage. Understanding the intricate relationship between cortisol and weight management is crucial, offering insights into both the challenges many face in achieving a healthy weight and potential strategies for navigating this complex interplay.

Cortisol: The Stress Hormone:

Cortisol, produced by the adrenal glands, is often dubbed the "stress hormone" due to its central role in the body's stress response. When confronted with a stressor, whether physical or psychological, the body releases cortisol as part of the adaptive mechanism designed to mobilize energy reserves for a rapid response. This acute stress response, commonly known as the "fight or flight" reaction, showcases cortisol's evolutionary significance in promoting survival.

However, the narrative evolves when stress becomes chronic, a prevalent feature of modern life. In a world marked by persistent stressors, from work pressures to personal challenges, cortisol can transition from a helpful ally to a potential foe. Prolonged elevation of cortisol levels is associated with a range of health issues, and its impact on weight management becomes a focal point of exploration.

Cortisol and Metabolism:

One of the key aspects of cortisol's influence on weight management lies in its impact on metabolism. In the acute stress response, cortisol mobilizes glucose and fatty acids, providing the body with a quick energy boost. This response is adaptive in situations that demand immediate action, such as escaping a perceived threat.

However, when stress is chronic, the persistent elevation of cortisol can lead to sustained mobilization of energy stores. This can result in increased levels of glucose in the bloodstream, potentially contributing to insulin resistance—a condition associated with weight gain and metabolic disorders. The intricate dance between cortisol and metabolism underscores the need for a nuanced understanding of how stress can influence body composition.

Appetite Regulation:

Cortisol's influence extends beyond metabolism to the complex realm of appetite regulation. In times of stress, cortisol interacts with the brain's appetite control centers, influencing food preferences and intake. For some individuals, stress may lead to increased cravings for high-calorie, comfort foods—often rich in sugars and fats. This behavioral response is thought to be an adaptive mechanism linked to the body's perceived need for quick energy during stressful situations.

The challenge arises when chronic stress perpetuates these cravings, contributing to unhealthy dietary patterns and potential weight gain. The intricate interplay between cortisol and appetite regulation sheds light on the behavioral aspects of weight management, emphasizing the importance of addressing not only dietary choices but also the underlying stressors that influence eating behaviors.

Fat Storage and Distribution:

Cortisol's impact on weight management also extends to its role in fat storage and distribution. Research suggests that elevated cortisol levels may contribute to the accumulation of visceral fat—fat stored around internal organs. Visceral fat is associated with an increased risk of metabolic disorders, including insulin resistance, type 2 diabetes, and cardiovascular issues.

The mechanisms through which cortisol influences fat distribution are complex and involve interactions with other hormones, such as insulin. Chronic elevation of cortisol can disrupt the delicate balance between hormones involved in fat metabolism, potentially favoring fat storage in the abdominal region. This visceral fat accumulation is not only a cosmetic concern but also a health risk, further emphasizing the need to understand and manage cortisol levels in the context of weight management.

Chronic Stress and Cortisol Dysregulation:

Central to the discussion of cortisol and weight management is the concept of chronic stress and cortisol dysregulation. Chronic stressors, whether related to work, relationships, or other life challenges, can lead to a persistent elevation of cortisol levels. This sustained presence of cortisol disrupts the delicate feedback loops that regulate the hormone's secretion and clearance.

Cortisol dysregulation is linked to a phenomenon known as "stress-induced obesity," where prolonged exposure to elevated cortisol contributes to weight gain, particularly around the abdominal area. The implications of this go beyond aesthetics, as abdominal obesity is associated with an increased risk of metabolic syndrome and cardiovascular diseases.

Moreover, chronic stress and cortisol dysregulation can create a vicious cycle. Weight gain itself can become a source of stress, further exacerbating cortisol levels and perpetuating unhealthy patterns of weight management. Breaking this cycle requires a holistic approach that addresses both the physiological and psychological aspects of stress and weight.

Strategies for Managing Cortisol and Promoting Healthy Weight Management:

1. Stress Reduction Techniques:

 - Mindfulness meditation, yoga, and deep breathing exercises are effective stress reduction techniques that have shown promise in lowering cortisol levels.

 - Incorporating regular breaks, leisure activities, and hobbies into daily routines can provide mental and emotional respite, helping to mitigate chronic stress.

2. Regular Exercise:

 - Physical activity is a powerful tool for managing cortisol levels. Regular exercise, whether aerobic or strength training, has been shown to reduce cortisol levels and improve overall well-being.

- Finding enjoyable forms of exercise can make it easier to incorporate physical activity into a routine, making it a sustainable aspect of weight management.

3. Adequate Sleep:

- Quality sleep is integral to cortisol regulation. Establishing a consistent sleep schedule, creating a conducive sleep environment, and practicing good sleep hygiene contribute to better sleep quality.

- Addressing sleep disturbances and disorders is crucial, as poor sleep can contribute to cortisol dysregulation and weight gain.

4. Balanced Nutrition:

- Adopting a balanced and nutritious diet plays a pivotal role in weight management and cortisol regulation. Nutrient-dense foods, rich in vitamins and minerals, support overall health and hormonal balance.

- Avoiding excessive consumption of refined sugars and processed foods can help stabilize blood sugar levels, reducing the potential impact of cortisol on metabolism.

5. Social Support and Connection:

- Cultivating social connections and building a support system can buffer the effects of stress. Positive social interactions and a strong support network contribute to emotional well-being, reducing the psychological impact of stressors.

6. Mindfulness and Cognitive Behavioral Techniques:

- Mindfulness-based interventions and cognitive-behavioral techniques can help individuals reframe their responses to stressors, fostering a more adaptive and resilient mindset.

- Developing coping strategies and problem-solving skills enhances the ability to navigate stressors without triggering prolonged cortisol release.

7. Professional Guidance:

- Seeking guidance from healthcare professionals, including nutritionists, psychologists, and endocrinologists, can provide personalized strategies for managing cortisol and achieving sustainable weight management goals.

- Medical evaluation can help identify underlying hormonal imbalances or health conditions that may contribute to weight-related challenges.

Conclusion:

In the intricate interplay between cortisol and weight management, a nuanced understanding emerges—one that recognizes the multifaceted nature of this relationship. Cortisol, as the stress hormone, responds dynamically to life's challenges, impacting metabolism, appetite regulation, and fat storage. While acute cortisol responses are adaptive, chronic stress can lead to dysregulation, contributing to weight-related challenges.

Addressing the complex connection between cortisol and weight management requires a holistic approach that encompasses both physiological and psychological dimensions. Strategies focused on stress reduction, regular exercise, adequate sleep, balanced nutrition, social support, and mindfulness offer a comprehensive toolkit for managing cortisol levels and promoting healthy weight management.

As individuals navigate the complexities of modern life, armed with knowledge and proactive measures, the narrative of cortisol's influence on weight management transforms from a potential obstacle to an opportunity for empowered, sustainable well-being. By unraveling the complex connection between cortisol and weight, individuals can embark on a journey towards achieving and maintaining a healthy weight while fostering resilience in the face of life's inevitable stressors.

Fertility and Cortisol Levels

The journey to parenthood is a profound and often intricate passage marked by numerous physiological and emotional nuances. In recent years, researchers and healthcare professionals have delved into the intricate interplay between fertility and cortisol levels—the primary stress hormone. Understanding how cortisol influences reproductive health is critical for those on the path to conception. This exploration not only sheds light on the physiological mechanisms at play but also offers insights into potential strategies for optimizing fertility in the context of cortisol dynamics.

The Cortisol Connection to Reproductive Health:

Cortisol, produced by the adrenal glands, is a central player in the body's stress response system. While the stress response, including the release of cortisol, is evolutionarily adaptive for short-term survival, chronic stress can disrupt various physiological processes, including those related to reproductive health.

In the context of fertility, cortisol's impact extends to the delicate balance of reproductive hormones, such as estrogen and progesterone, which are crucial for menstrual cycle regulation and ovulation. Chronic stress, and the resulting elevation of cortisol levels, can potentially interfere with this delicate hormonal balance, creating challenges for those trying to conceive.

Ovulation Disruption:

One key aspect of fertility influenced by cortisol is the process of ovulation. Ovulation, the release of a mature egg from the ovary, is a fundamental step in conception. The intricate dance of hormones, including luteinizing hormone (LH) and follicle-stimulating hormone (FSH), orchestrates this process. However, elevated cortisol levels, particularly over an extended period, may disrupt this delicate hormonal symphony.

Research suggests that chronic stress can lead to irregularities in menstrual cycles, affecting the timing and regularity of ovulation. This irregularity may present a significant obstacle for those trying to conceive, as accurate prediction of fertile windows becomes challenging. Understanding the impact of cortisol on ovulation provides a crucial perspective for individuals and couples navigating fertility challenges.

Impact on Reproductive Hormones:

Cortisol's influence on fertility extends beyond its effects on ovulation to its impact on key reproductive hormones. Chronic stress may alter the production and regulation of hormones such as estrogen and progesterone, which play pivotal roles in the menstrual cycle and the implantation of a fertilized egg.

Elevated cortisol levels can disrupt the normal pulsatile release of gonadotropin-releasing hormone (GnRH) from the hypothalamus, leading to imbalances in FSH and LH release from the pituitary gland. This disruption can, in turn, affect ovarian function and the development of healthy eggs. Additionally, cortisol may directly impact the ovaries, influencing the production of sex hormones and potentially impairing the overall reproductive process.

Understanding these intricate hormonal interactions is essential for individuals and couples seeking to optimize their fertility. It emphasizes the need to address not only the physical aspects of conception but also the underlying stressors that may impact hormonal balance.

Implantation and Pregnancy:

The journey from fertilization to a successful pregnancy involves a series of complex steps, and cortisol's influence extends to the critical phase of embryo implantation. Elevated cortisol levels have been associated with changes in the endometrial environment—the lining of the uterus—which may affect the receptivity of the uterus for implantation.

Moreover, chronic stress and cortisol dysregulation may contribute to inflammation and immune system imbalances that can impact the implantation process. This highlights the interconnectedness of the stress response, hormonal balance, and the intricate processes involved in early pregnancy.

Male Fertility and Cortisol:

While much of the focus has been on cortisol's impact on female fertility, it's crucial to acknowledge its potential effects on male fertility as well. Cortisol dysregulation can influence the quality and quantity of sperm, potentially contributing to male infertility.

Elevated cortisol levels may lead to changes in testosterone production and disrupt the delicate hormonal balance necessary for spermatogenesis—the process of sperm development. Understanding the impact of stress on male reproductive health underscores the importance of a holistic approach to fertility that considers both partners.

Strategies for Managing Cortisol and Optimizing Fertility:

1. Stress Reduction Techniques:

   - Mindfulness-based stress reduction (MBSR), yoga, and meditation have shown promise in reducing cortisol levels and promoting emotional well-being.

   - Incorporating stress reduction techniques into daily life can be particularly beneficial for couples navigating the emotional challenges of fertility.

2. Regular Exercise:

- Physical activity has been linked to lower cortisol levels and improved fertility outcomes. Moderate exercise, such as walking or swimming, can contribute to overall well-being.

- Finding enjoyable forms of exercise not only supports stress reduction but also promotes a healthy lifestyle conducive to fertility.

3. Adequate Sleep:

- Quality sleep is integral to cortisol regulation. Establishing a consistent sleep routine and addressing sleep disturbances are essential for optimizing fertility.

- Sleep hygiene practices, such as creating a conducive sleep environment and avoiding electronic devices before bedtime, contribute to better sleep quality.

4. Nutrient-Rich Diet:

- Adopting a balanced and nutrient-dense diet is vital for overall health and hormonal balance. Including foods rich in antioxidants, vitamins, and minerals supports reproductive health.

- Avoiding excessive caffeine and alcohol consumption, which can impact cortisol levels and fertility, is advisable for individuals seeking to conceive.

5. Counseling and Support:

- Seeking counseling or support groups can be beneficial for couples facing fertility challenges. Addressing the emotional aspects of infertility and finding healthy coping mechanisms contribute to overall well-being.

- Professional guidance from fertility specialists or reproductive endocrinologists can provide personalized insights into the specific factors influencing fertility and potential interventions.

6. Mind-Body Interventions:

- Mind-body interventions, including guided imagery, relaxation techniques, and acupuncture, have been explored for their potential to positively influence fertility outcomes.

- These interventions focus on the interconnectedness of mind and body, aiming to create a supportive environment for conception.

7. Medical Evaluation:

- If fertility challenges persist, seeking a medical evaluation is crucial. Hormonal assessments, fertility testing, and consultations with reproductive specialists can provide a comprehensive understanding of potential factors influencing fertility.

- Medical interventions, such as assisted reproductive technologies (ART) or hormone therapies, may be recommended based on individual circumstances.

Conclusion:

The intersection of fertility and cortisol levels underscores the intricate interplay between stress and reproductive health. While cortisol, as the stress hormone, is a natural and adaptive part of the body's response to challenges, chronic stress can disrupt hormonal balance and potentially impact fertility.

Understanding the nuances of cortisol's influence on ovulation, reproductive hormones, and the implantation process provides valuable insights for individuals and couples navigating the path to conception. Moreover, recognizing the potential impact of stress on both female and male fertility emphasizes the importance of a holistic approach that addresses the physical, emotional, and lifestyle factors influencing reproductive health.

As we delve into the complexities of fertility and cortisol levels, a narrative of empowerment emerges—one that encourages proactive measures, emotional well-being, and informed choices. By integrating stress-reduction strategies, healthy lifestyle practices, and seeking professional guidance when needed, individuals and couples can optimize their chances for a healthy and successful fertility journey. In this exploration, the integration of mind and body becomes paramount, fostering an environment conducive to the creation of new life.

Navigating Menopause: Cortisol's Influence

Menopause, a natural and inevitable phase in a woman's life, marks the end of reproductive capacity and the onset of profound hormonal changes. While estrogen and progesterone shifts are well-known players in this transition, the influence of cortisol, the primary stress hormone, often takes a backstage. This exploration aims to unravel the intricate connection between cortisol and menopause, shedding light on how stress and cortisol dynamics contribute to the complexities experienced during this transformative period.

Menopause and Hormonal Dynamics:

Menopause typically occurs between the ages of 45 and 55, signaling the cessation of menstrual cycles and the end of fertility. The primary hormonal players during this transition are estrogen and progesterone, whose levels decline as the ovaries reduce their production. The resultant hormonal fluctuations give rise to various physical and psychological symptoms, ranging from hot flashes and night sweats to mood swings and sleep disturbances.

While estrogen and progesterone changes are central to menopausal symptoms, the interplay with cortisol adds another layer of complexity. Cortisol, produced by the adrenal glands, plays a crucial role in the body's stress response. As women navigate the challenges of menopause, the impact of stress on cortisol dynamics becomes a significant factor influencing the overall experience.

Stress, Cortisol, and Menopausal Symptoms:

Chronic stress, a prevalent aspect of modern lifestyles, can contribute to heightened cortisol levels. The intricate relationship between stress and cortisol becomes particularly relevant during menopause, as cortisol interacts with hormonal changes and exacerbates certain symptoms.

1. Hot Flashes and Night Sweats:

   - Stress-induced cortisol release may trigger or intensify hot flashes and night sweats, common and disruptive symptoms during menopause.

   - The body's stress response, characterized by cortisol surges, can contribute to the dilation of blood vessels and increased body temperature, amplifying the frequency and intensity of these episodes.

2. Mood Swings and Anxiety:

   - Cortisol, when chronically elevated, can impact neurotransmitters and contribute to mood swings and increased anxiety levels.

   - The emotional roller coaster experienced by many women during menopause may be influenced by the intricate interplay between cortisol and hormonal changes.

3. Sleep Disturbances:

   - Elevated cortisol levels, especially during nighttime, can disrupt sleep patterns. Cortisol's role in the body's natural circadian rhythm may contribute to insomnia or fragmented sleep.

   - Sleep disturbances are a common complaint during menopause, and the influence of cortisol adds a layer of complexity to the understanding of sleep challenges.

4. Weight Changes:

   - Cortisol's impact on metabolism and fat storage can contribute to weight changes during menopause. Stress-induced cortisol release may lead to abdominal fat accumulation.

   - Women experiencing weight changes during menopause may benefit from addressing both hormonal shifts and stress-related factors influencing cortisol dynamics.

The Role of Cortisol in Hormonal Balance:

Beyond exacerbating menopausal symptoms, cortisol's influence extends to hormonal balance and the regulation of sex hormones, including estrogen. Chronic stress can disrupt the delicate equilibrium of the hypothalamic-pituitary-adrenal (HPA) axis, affecting the production and regulation of hormones.

1. Estrogen and Cortisol Interaction:

   - Cortisol competes with other hormones, including estrogen, for binding sites on receptors. Elevated cortisol levels may interfere with the normal functioning of estrogen.

   - This interplay can contribute to imbalances in hormonal ratios, potentially impacting the severity and duration of menopausal symptoms.

2. Bone Health:

   - Cortisol dynamics are intricately linked to bone metabolism. Chronic elevation of cortisol is associated with decreased bone density and increased risk of osteoporosis.

   - Considering the decline in estrogen levels during menopause, the additional impact of cortisol on bone health becomes a critical aspect to address for overall well-being.

Strategies for Cortisol Management during Menopause:

1. Stress Reduction Techniques:

   - Incorporating stress reduction techniques, such as mindfulness meditation, deep breathing exercises, and yoga, can help manage cortisol levels.

- Regular practice of these techniques provides women with effective tools to navigate the emotional and physiological challenges of menopause.

2. Regular Exercise:

- Physical activity is a natural stress reliever and can contribute to cortisol regulation. Engaging in regular exercise, whether aerobic or strength training, promotes overall well-being during menopause.

- Finding enjoyable forms of exercise not only supports stress reduction but also contributes to maintaining bone density and managing weight.

3. Adequate Sleep:

- Prioritizing quality sleep is crucial for cortisol regulation and overall health during menopause. Establishing a consistent sleep routine and creating a conducive sleep environment are essential.

- Addressing sleep disturbances promptly supports women in managing cortisol-related challenges and optimizing their well-being.

4. Nutrient-Rich Diet:

- Adopting a balanced and nutrient-dense diet supports hormonal balance and overall health during menopause. Foods rich in antioxidants, vitamins, and minerals contribute to stress resilience.

- Limiting the intake of stimulants, such as caffeine and refined sugars, helps stabilize blood sugar levels and may positively influence cortisol dynamics.

5. Social Support:

- Cultivating strong social connections and seeking support from friends, family, or support groups can be invaluable during menopause.

- Social support buffers the impact of stress, fostering emotional well-being and contributing to cortisol management.

6. Mind-Body Practices:

- Mind-body practices, including acupuncture, guided imagery, and biofeedback, have shown promise in managing cortisol levels and improving overall menopausal symptoms.

- Integrating these practices into a holistic approach to well-being provides women with additional tools for navigating the challenges of menopause.

7. Professional Guidance:

- Seeking guidance from healthcare professionals, including gynecologists, endocrinologists, or mental health professionals, can provide personalized insights into managing menopausal symptoms and cortisol dynamics.

- Hormone replacement therapy (HRT) may be considered under the guidance of a healthcare provider to address specific hormonal imbalances.

Empowering Women through Cortisol Awareness:

As women traverse the uncharted territory of menopause, understanding cortisol's influence becomes a powerful tool for empowerment. Recognizing the impact of stress on menopausal symptoms and hormonal balance allows women to make informed choices and adopt strategies that promote both physical and emotional well-being.

Embracing a holistic approach that addresses stressors, incorporates healthy lifestyle practices, and seeks support when needed fosters resilience during this transformative phase. By navigating menopause with a nuanced understanding of cortisol's role, women can reclaim agency over their well-being, embracing the journey with grace and resilience.

In essence, menopause is not solely a culmination but a transition—an opportunity for women to navigate change with wisdom and self-care. Cortisol, with its intricate influence, becomes not just a physiological factor but a guidepost in this transformative journey, encouraging women to approach menopause with knowledge, resilience, and a commitment to holistic well-being.

Longevity and the Cortisol Connection

Longevity, the pursuit of a longer and healthier life, has intrigued humanity for centuries. In this quest, the role of cortisol, the primary stress hormone, emerges as a significant factor influencing the aging process. As we unravel the cortisol connection to longevity, we delve into the complex interplay between stress, cortisol dynamics, and the intricate mechanisms that govern the aging of the human body.

Understanding Cortisol's Role in the Stress Response:

Cortisol, produced by the adrenal glands, is a pivotal player in the body's stress response system. When faced with a stressor, whether physical or psychological, cortisol levels surge, initiating a cascade of physiological changes. This acute stress response is designed to mobilize energy reserves, sharpen cognitive functions, and prepare the body for immediate action—an adaptive mechanism finely tuned by evolution.

However, the intricacies of cortisol's influence become apparent when stress becomes chronic. In the modern landscape, characterized by persistent stressors and a frenetic pace of life, cortisol may linger in the bloodstream for extended periods. This chronic elevation of cortisol is associated with a range of health implications, influencing not only immediate stress responses but also long-term processes linked to aging.

Cortisol and Cellular Aging:

At the cellular level, the impact of cortisol on aging is profound. Telomeres, protective caps at the ends of chromosomes, play a crucial role in maintaining genomic stability. As cells divide, telomeres naturally shorten, eventually leading to cell senescence or programmed cell death. Chronic stress and elevated cortisol levels have been linked to accelerated telomere shortening, suggesting a potential mechanism through which stress influences cellular aging.

Moreover, cortisol's influence extends to the intricate world of epigenetics—the modifications that affect gene expression without altering the underlying DNA sequence. Stress-induced changes in DNA methylation and histone modification patterns have been associated with accelerated aging processes. Understanding these molecular mechanisms provides insights into how cortisol, as a mediator of stress, may contribute to the aging of cells and tissues.

Cortisol, Inflammation, and Aging:

Inflammation, a natural response to injury or infection, plays a dual role in the aging process. While acute inflammation is a protective mechanism, chronic inflammation is implicated in various age-related diseases. Cortisol, as a regulator of the immune system, exerts both anti-inflammatory and pro-inflammatory effects, depending on the context.

Chronic stress and cortisol dysregulation can tip the balance toward a pro-inflammatory state. This chronic low-grade inflammation, often referred to as "inflammaging," contributes to the aging of tissues and organs. The link between cortisol, inflammation, and aging emphasizes the importance of stress management in promoting not only longevity but also a healthy and resilient aging process.

Cortisol and Hormonal Decline:

Hormonal decline is a hallmark of the aging process, and cortisol's influence intersects with the regulation of other hormones. The delicate balance between cortisol and hormones such as dehydroepiandrosterone (DHEA), a precursor to sex hormones, becomes disrupted with age. This imbalance can contribute to the symptoms associated with aging, such as reduced bone density, muscle mass, and cognitive function.

Furthermore, cortisol's interaction with insulin, the hormone regulating blood sugar levels, influences metabolic health. Chronic stress and elevated cortisol levels are associated with insulin resistance—a condition linked to diabetes and other age-related metabolic disorders. Managing cortisol becomes integral to preserving hormonal balance and promoting overall health as individuals age.

The Impact of Chronic Stress on Cognitive Aging:

Cortisol's influence on cognitive function is a significant aspect of the cortisol connection to aging. Chronic stress and prolonged cortisol elevation have been associated with structural and functional changes in the brain. The hippocampus, a region critical for memory and learning, is particularly susceptible to the effects of cortisol.

Research suggests that chronic stress may lead to hippocampal atrophy—a reduction in the size of the hippocampus—and impairments in neurogenesis, the process of generating new neurons. These changes are implicated in age-related cognitive decline and neurodegenerative diseases such as Alzheimer's. The cortisol connection to cognitive aging underscores the importance of stress management in preserving cognitive function throughout the lifespan.

Strategies for Managing Cortisol and Promoting Longevity:

1. Stress Reduction Techniques:

- Incorporating stress reduction techniques into daily life is pivotal for managing cortisol levels. Mindfulness meditation, deep breathing exercises, and progressive muscle relaxation are effective tools for stress reduction.

- Establishing a regular practice of these techniques contributes not only to immediate stress relief but also to long-term resilience.

2. Regular Exercise:

- Physical activity is a natural stress reliever and contributes to cortisol regulation. Regular exercise, whether aerobic or strength training, promotes overall well-being and supports healthy aging.

- Engaging in enjoyable forms of exercise enhances adherence to a routine, making it a sustainable lifestyle choice.

3. Adequate Sleep:

- Quality sleep is integral to cortisol regulation and overall health. Establishing a consistent sleep routine, creating a conducive sleep environment, and addressing sleep disturbances contribute to better sleep quality.

- Prioritizing sleep as a crucial component of a longevity-focused lifestyle supports both physical and cognitive health.

4. Nutrient-Rich Diet:

- Adopting a balanced and nutrient-dense diet supports overall health and hormonal balance. Antioxidant-rich foods, omega-3 fatty acids, and a variety of fruits and vegetables contribute to stress resilience and inflammation management.

- Limiting the intake of processed foods, sugars, and excessive caffeine supports metabolic health and promotes longevity.

5. Social Connections:

- Cultivating strong social connections and maintaining a supportive social network contribute to emotional well-being and stress management.

- Regular social interactions, whether in-person or virtual, provide a buffer against the negative effects of chronic stress and contribute to a sense of purpose and belonging.

6. Mind-Body Practices:

- Mind-body practices, including yoga, tai chi, and qigong, combine physical movement with mindfulness, promoting both physical and mental well-being.

- Integrating mind-body practices into a longevity-focused lifestyle enhances flexibility, balance, and emotional resilience.

7. Professional Guidance:

- Seeking guidance from healthcare professionals, including endocrinologists, nutritionists, and mental health professionals, can provide personalized insights into managing cortisol and promoting longevity.

- Hormone replacement therapy (HRT) or other medical interventions may be considered under the guidance of healthcare providers based on individual health needs.

Conclusion:

In the intricate tapestry of longevity, the cortisol connection emerges as a significant thread—a dynamic interplay between stress, hormones, and the aging process. Cortisol's influence on cellular aging, inflammation, hormonal decline, and cognitive function underscores its pivotal role in shaping the trajectory of aging.

As individuals embark on the journey toward a longer and healthier life, understanding and managing cortisol dynamics become essential components of a holistic approach to longevity. The integration of stress reduction strategies, lifestyle choices, and a supportive social environment empowers individuals to age gracefully and resiliently.

The cortisol connection to longevity invites a paradigm shift—one that acknowledges the impact of stress on the aging process while highlighting the potential for proactive measures to promote healthy aging. By navigating the complexities of cortisol's influence with knowledge and intention, individuals can embrace the pursuit of longevity with a sense of empowerment, resilience, and a commitment to nurturing a vibrant and fulfilling life.

Stress and Cortisol

In the intricate dance of human biology, stress and cortisol emerge as central players, intricately linked in the body's response to challenges. Stress, whether triggered by external events or internal pressures, sets off a cascade of physiological reactions, with cortisol, often referred to as the "stress hormone," at the forefront. This exploration delves into the multifaceted relationship between stress and cortisol, unraveling the physiological mechanisms, the impact on health, and strategies for managing this intricate interplay.

The Stress Response: A Evolutionary Legacy:

The stress response, often dubbed the "fight or flight" reaction, is deeply rooted in human evolution. When faced with a perceived threat, the body mobilizes resources to prepare for rapid action. This adaptive mechanism, honed over millennia, involves the activation of the sympathetic nervous system and the release of stress hormones, including cortisol.

In the face of acute stress, cortisol orchestrates a series of responses aimed at enhancing immediate survival. It prompts the release of glucose into the bloodstream, providing a quick energy boost. Simultaneously, it redirects resources away from non-essential functions, such as digestion and immune response, toward processes crucial for survival in the moment.

While this acute stress response is a survival advantage in situations requiring swift action, the challenge arises in the context of modern life. Chronic stress, stemming from factors such as work pressures, financial worries, or interpersonal conflicts, can sustain elevated cortisol levels, triggering a cascade of physiological changes that have far-reaching implications for health.

Cortisol: The Body's Stress Messenger:

Cortisol, produced by the adrenal glands, is a steroid hormone that serves as a messenger between the stress response system and various tissues in the body. Its release is intricately regulated by the hypothalamus-pituitary-adrenal (HPA) axis—a complex feedback system that maintains the delicate balance of cortisol in circulation.

Upon encountering a stressor, the hypothalamus releases corticotropin-releasing hormone (CRH), which signals the pituitary gland to release adrenocorticotropic hormone (ACTH). ACTH, in turn, stimulates the adrenal glands to produce and release cortisol. This finely tuned system ensures a rapid and precise response to stressors.

Cortisol Dynamics: From Peaks to Rhythms:

Cortisol levels in the body follow a circadian rhythm, with a natural peak in the early morning to help kickstart the day and a gradual decline throughout the day. This rhythmic pattern is crucial for various physiological processes, including metabolism, immune function, and the sleep-wake cycle.

However, chronic stress can disrupt this natural rhythm. Prolonged elevation of cortisol levels, especially when the stress response is activated frequently, can lead to dysregulation of the HPA axis. This dysregulation is associated with a host of health issues, from metabolic disorders and immune suppression to cognitive impairments and mental health challenges.

Impact of Chronic Stress and Elevated Cortisol:

1. Metabolic Effects:

   - Cortisol plays a central role in glucose metabolism, promoting the release of glucose into the bloodstream for quick energy. In the context of chronic stress, this mechanism can contribute to elevated blood sugar levels.

   - Prolonged exposure to elevated cortisol is associated with insulin resistance, a condition where cells become less responsive to insulin, potentially leading to type 2 diabetes and metabolic syndrome.

2. Immune System Suppression:

   - While cortisol is anti-inflammatory in nature, chronic elevation can suppress the immune system. This makes individuals more susceptible to infections and hinders the body's ability to mount an effective immune response.

   - Long-term immune suppression contributes to a higher risk of illnesses, including respiratory infections and autoimmune disorders.

3. Cognitive Impact:

   - Cortisol's influence on the brain extends to various cognitive functions. In acute stress, cortisol enhances memory formation and alertness.

   - However, chronic stress can impair cognitive function, particularly memory and concentration. It is associated with structural changes in the hippocampus, a brain region crucial for memory and learning.

4. Cardiovascular Effects:

   - Elevated cortisol levels can contribute to hypertension (high blood pressure) and cardiovascular disease. Cortisol's impact on blood vessel constriction and inflammation plays a role in these cardiovascular effects.

   - Chronic stress and cortisol dysregulation are recognized as risk factors for heart disease and may contribute to the development of atherosclerosis.

5. Mental Health Challenges:

- The intricate interplay between chronic stress, cortisol, and mental health is well-documented. Persistent elevation of cortisol is associated with an increased risk of mood disorders, including anxiety and depression.

- Cortisol dysregulation can also impact the function of neurotransmitters, such as serotonin and dopamine, further contributing to mental health challenges.

Strategies for Managing Stress and Cortisol:

1. Mindfulness and Relaxation Techniques:

- Mindfulness meditation, deep breathing exercises, and progressive muscle relaxation are effective tools for managing stress and lowering cortisol levels.

- Incorporating these practices into daily routines can promote a sense of calm and resilience in the face of stressors.

2. Regular Exercise:

- Physical activity is a natural stress reliever and can contribute to cortisol regulation. Engaging in regular exercise, whether aerobic or strength training, promotes overall well-being.

- Finding enjoyable forms of exercise makes it more likely to become a consistent part of one's routine.

3. Adequate Sleep:

- Quality sleep is integral to cortisol regulation and overall health. Establishing a consistent sleep routine, creating a conducive sleep environment, and addressing sleep disturbances contribute to better sleep quality.

- Prioritizing sleep is crucial for allowing the body to recover and maintain a healthy cortisol rhythm.

4. Balanced Nutrition:

- Adopting a balanced and nutrient-dense diet supports overall health and cortisol regulation. Nutrient-rich foods, including fruits, vegetables, and whole grains, provide essential vitamins and minerals.

- Avoiding excessive caffeine and refined sugars helps stabilize blood sugar levels and prevent additional stress on the body.

5. Social Support:

- Cultivating strong social connections and seeking support from friends, family, or support groups can be invaluable for managing stress.

- Social support acts as a buffer against the negative effects of chronic stress, promoting emotional well-being.

6. Time Management:

- Effectively managing time and setting realistic goals can reduce the perception of stressors. Breaking tasks into smaller, manageable steps can make them feel more achievable.

- Prioritizing and delegating tasks when possible helps prevent feelings of overwhelm.

7. Professional Support:

- Seeking guidance from mental health professionals, such as psychologists or counselors, can provide strategies for coping with stress and improving resilience.

- For individuals facing chronic stress and cortisol-related health issues, consulting with healthcare professionals, including endocrinologists, may be necessary for a comprehensive assessment and personalized recommendations.

Conclusion:

The link between stress and cortisol is a dynamic and intricate dance that influences numerous aspects of health and well-being. While stress is an inevitable part of life, understanding the impact of chronic stress and elevated cortisol levels provides a foundation for proactive management.

Empowering individuals with effective strategies for stress reduction, lifestyle modifications, and social support fosters resilience in the face of life's challenges. By unraveling the link between stress and cortisol, individuals can navigate their daily lives with a heightened awareness of the intricate interplay between mind and body, ultimately promoting a state of well-being and balance.

Interplay Between the Gut Microbiome and Cortisol

In recent years, scientific exploration has increasingly delved into the intricate relationship between the gut microbiome and various aspects of human health. One particularly fascinating avenue of research has focused on the interplay between the gut microbiome and cortisol, the primary hormone associated with the body's stress response. This dynamic interaction between the gut and stress hormones opens new avenues for understanding how our internal ecosystems influence not only digestive health but also broader physiological and psychological well-being.

The gut microbiome, a diverse community of trillions of microorganisms residing in the gastrointestinal tract, plays a crucial role in maintaining health and supporting various bodily functions. Comprising bacteria, viruses, fungi, and other microbes, this complex ecosystem forms a symbiotic relationship with the human host, influencing processes ranging from digestion to

immune function. Recent advancements in technology have enabled scientists to unravel the intricate web of interactions between these microorganisms and the host's physiological systems.

Cortisol, often dubbed the "stress hormone," is produced by the adrenal glands in response to stressors. Its primary role is to mobilize energy reserves, sharpen focus, and prepare the body for a fight-or-flight response. While cortisol is essential for survival in acute stress situations, chronic elevation can have detrimental effects on health. Beyond its role in stress response, cortisol also plays a role in metabolism, immune function, and the regulation of blood pressure.

The gut-brain axis, a bidirectional communication network between the gut and the central nervous system, serves as a crucial link in understanding the relationship between the gut microbiome and cortisol. This intricate connection involves various signaling pathways, including the nervous system, immune system, and endocrine system. Emerging research suggests that the gut microbiome actively participates in this axis, influencing not only digestive health but also cognitive function and stress responses.

In laboratory studies, researchers have observed the fascinating ability of gut microbes to influence stress hormones, including cortisol. Animal studies, particularly in rodents, have provided valuable insights into the impact of the gut microbiome on the HPA (hypothalamic-pituitary-adrenal) axis, the central regulator of cortisol release.

A landmark study published in the journal "Psychoneuroendocrinology" demonstrated that germ-free mice, devoid of gut microbiota, exhibited altered stress responses compared to their conventionally raised counterparts. The germ-free mice displayed exaggerated release of stress hormones, including cortisol, in response to stressors. This finding indicated that the presence or absence of gut microbes could modulate the physiological response to stress.

The gut microbiome's influence on stress hormones extends beyond the direct modulation of cortisol. Gut microbes actively participate in the production and regulation of neurotransmitters and other hormones that play a role in mood and stress. For instance, certain bacteria in the gut contribute to the synthesis of neurotransmitters like serotonin, often referred to as the "feel-good" neurotransmitter.

Moreover, the gut microbiome produces metabolites, such as short-chain fatty acids (SCFAs), that can influence the activity of the HPA axis. SCFAs, generated through the fermentation of dietary fiber by gut bacteria, have been shown to have anti-inflammatory and neuroprotective effects. These microbial byproducts can interact with immune cells and neural pathways, ultimately impacting the regulation of cortisol.

Dysbiosis, an imbalance in the composition and diversity of the gut microbiome, has been linked to various health issues, including mental health disorders and dysregulation of stress hormones. In conditions where dysbiosis is prevalent, alterations in the microbial community may contribute to an overactive stress response and cortisol dysregulation.

Chronic stress itself can induce dysbiosis, creating a feedback loop where stress disrupts the gut microbiome, and the altered microbiome, in turn, contributes to heightened stress responses. This

bidirectional relationship underscores the importance of maintaining a balanced gut microbiome for overall stress resilience.

The therapeutic potential of modulating the gut microbiome for cortisol regulation has led to investigations into the use of prebiotics and probiotics. Prebiotics, non-digestible fibers that nourish beneficial gut bacteria, and probiotics, live microorganisms with health benefits, are being explored for their ability to support a balanced and resilient gut microbiome.

Research in both animals and humans suggests that certain probiotic strains, such as those belonging to the Lactobacillus and Bifidobacterium genera, may have stress-reducing effects. These probiotics may influence the gut-brain axis, promoting the production of anti-inflammatory compounds and modulating the HPA axis to regulate cortisol release.

Beyond microbial interventions, lifestyle factors play a pivotal role in shaping the gut microbiome and influencing cortisol levels. Diet, exercise, and sleep patterns, known as the pillars of a healthy lifestyle, have profound impacts on both the gut microbiome composition and the stress response.

A diet rich in fiber from diverse plant sources supports microbial diversity and the production of beneficial metabolites. Conversely, a diet high in processed foods and sugars may contribute to dysbiosis and inflammation, potentially influencing cortisol regulation.

Regular exercise has been associated with a more diverse and balanced gut microbiome. Additionally, exercise can have direct effects on cortisol regulation, promoting a healthier stress response.

Adequate and restful sleep is crucial for maintaining a resilient stress response and supporting a balanced gut microbiome. Disruptions in sleep patterns have been linked to alterations in cortisol levels.

While our understanding of the intricate link between the gut microbiome and cortisol is rapidly evolving, several questions remain unanswered. Future research may explore the specific mechanisms through which gut microbes communicate with the HPA axis and the potential for targeted interventions to modulate cortisol in various health conditions.

The implications of this research extend beyond stress management. Given the systemic effects of cortisol on metabolism, immune function, and mental health, a balanced gut microbiome emerges as a key player in promoting overall well-being.

In unraveling the complex connection between the gut microbiome and cortisol, science is uncovering a harmonious symphony within our bodies. The interplay between gut microbes and stress hormones is a dynamic dance that influences not only digestive health but also our responses to the myriad stressors of life.

As we embrace the potential therapeutic avenues presented by prebiotics, probiotics, and lifestyle modifications, the concept of "mind-gut health" takes center stage. A holistic approach to well-being involves nurturing both the gut microbiome and the delicate balance of stress hormones, ultimately contributing to a resilient and thriving body and mind. The ongoing exploration of this

intricate relationship promises a future where personalized interventions harness the power of the gut microbiome to enhance stress resilience and promote optimal health.

Chapter Three

Lifestyle Strategies for Cortisol Regulation

In the hustle and bustle of modern life, where stressors seem to be constant companions, understanding and managing cortisol levels become integral to maintaining overall health and well-being. Cortisol, the primary stress hormone, plays a crucial role in the body's response to stress, and chronic elevation can have far-reaching implications. This exploration delves into lifestyle strategies aimed at regulating cortisol, offering practical insights into fostering balance, resilience, and a healthier relationship with stress in the contemporary landscape.

1. Mindfulness and Stress Reduction Techniques:

Mindfulness meditation, deep breathing exercises, and progressive muscle relaxation are potent tools for cultivating a sense of calm and regulating cortisol levels. Engaging in mindfulness practices involves bringing focused attention to the present moment, creating a buffer against the anxiety-inducing effects of chronic stress.

Mindfulness practices encourage a non-judgmental awareness of thoughts and sensations, helping individuals respond to stressors with greater clarity and composure. The meditative aspect of these practices has been shown to lower cortisol levels and promote a more balanced stress response.

Incorporating brief mindfulness sessions into daily routines, whether during breaks at work or before bedtime, can contribute to overall stress reduction and cortisol regulation.

2. Regular Physical Activity:

Physical exercise is a natural antidote to stress and a key player in cortisol regulation. Engaging in regular aerobic exercise, such as jogging, swimming, or cycling, helps dissipate accumulated stress and prompts the release of endorphins, the body's natural mood elevators.

Moreover, strength training exercises contribute to cortisol regulation by promoting a balanced hormonal response. Building and maintaining muscle mass through resistance training can enhance the body's ability to manage stress and maintain a healthy cortisol rhythm.

Striking a balance between cardiovascular exercise and strength training offers comprehensive benefits for both physical and mental well-being, contributing to an overall healthier stress response.

3. Adequate Sleep Hygiene:

Quality sleep is a cornerstone of cortisol regulation. Establishing a consistent sleep routine and prioritizing sufficient hours of restful sleep each night are essential for maintaining a healthy circadian rhythm.

Cortisol follows a natural circadian pattern, peaking in the early morning to help wake the body and gradually declining throughout the day. Disruptions to this rhythm, often caused by inadequate sleep or irregular sleep patterns, can lead to cortisol dysregulation.

Practices such as creating a comfortable sleep environment, avoiding electronic devices before bedtime, and maintaining a regular sleep schedule contribute to improved sleep quality and support cortisol balance.

4. Balanced Nutrition:

Nutrient-dense and balanced eating habits play a crucial role in cortisol regulation. Adopting a diet rich in whole foods, including fruits, vegetables, lean proteins, and whole grains, provides the body with the necessary nutrients to function optimally.

Excessive consumption of refined sugars, processed foods, and caffeine can contribute to fluctuations in blood sugar levels and trigger cortisol release. On the other hand, a balanced diet with adequate fiber, vitamins, and minerals helps stabilize blood sugar, reducing the strain on the body's stress response system.

Hydration is another important aspect of nutrition. Maintaining adequate fluid intake supports overall health and helps the body manage stress more efficiently.

5. Social Support and Connection:

Building and nurturing social connections is a powerful strategy for cortisol regulation. Meaningful relationships and a strong support system act as buffers against the negative effects of chronic stress.

Spending time with friends and family, engaging in social activities, and participating in community events foster a sense of belonging and emotional support. Social interactions trigger the release of oxytocin, a hormone that counters the effects of cortisol and promotes a sense of calm.

In times of stress, having a network of supportive individuals provides avenues for sharing concerns, seeking advice, and receiving emotional reassurance. Strong social connections contribute not only to cortisol regulation but also to overall mental and emotional well-being.

6. Time Management and Prioritization:

The demands of a fast-paced lifestyle can contribute to chronic stress, leading to sustained cortisol elevation. Effective time management and prioritization are valuable skills for navigating daily responsibilities without succumbing to overwhelming stressors.

Breaking tasks into smaller, more manageable steps, setting realistic goals, and learning to delegate when necessary contribute to a more balanced approach to time management. This, in turn, helps prevent a constant state of heightened stress and supports cortisol regulation.

Establishing clear boundaries between work and personal life, setting aside time for relaxation and leisure activities, and recognizing the importance of downtime all contribute to a healthier lifestyle and cortisol balance.

7. Mindful Nutrition and Hydration:

In addition to a balanced diet, paying attention to mindful eating and staying adequately hydrated are essential components of cortisol regulation. Mindful eating involves being present and fully engaged in the eating experience, which can positively impact digestion and nutrient absorption.

Avoiding excessive caffeine intake, especially in the later part of the day, is crucial for preventing disruptions to sleep patterns and cortisol rhythms. While moderate caffeine consumption may have its benefits, excessive reliance on caffeinated beverages can contribute to an overactive stress response.

Hydration, on the other hand, supports various physiological functions, including cortisol regulation. Drinking an adequate amount of water throughout the day helps maintain overall health and contributes to the body's ability to manage stress.

8. Leisure and Relaxation Activities:

Incorporating leisure and relaxation activities into daily life is vital for promoting cortisol balance. Engaging in activities that bring joy, relaxation, and a sense of fulfillment contributes to overall well-being.

Hobbies, reading, listening to music, spending time in nature, and practicing art or creativity are examples of leisure activities that help shift the focus away from stressors and provide an opportunity for rejuvenation. These activities contribute to a more balanced cortisol response by promoting a positive emotional state.

9. Cognitive and Emotional Wellness Practices:

The mind-body connection is evident in the intricate relationship between cognitive and emotional well-being and cortisol regulation. Mind-body practices, such as mindfulness-based stress reduction (MBSR), guided imagery, and cognitive-behavioral therapy (CBT), offer tools for managing stress at the cognitive and emotional levels.

These practices involve cultivating awareness of thought patterns, challenging negative beliefs, and developing healthier ways of coping with stress. By addressing stressors at their cognitive roots, individuals can influence the body's physiological response, including cortisol release.

10. Seeking Professional Guidance:

In cases where chronic stress and cortisol dysregulation persist despite lifestyle efforts, seeking professional guidance is crucial. Healthcare professionals, including endocrinologists, psychologists, and nutritionists, can provide personalized assessments and recommendations.

Medical professionals may conduct tests to assess cortisol levels, hormonal balance, and overall health. Based on the results, they can offer targeted interventions, which may include dietary adjustments, stress management techniques, and, in some cases, medications or hormone therapies.

Conclusion:

Navigating the intricate web of stress and cortisol regulation requires a multifaceted approach that encompasses various aspects of lifestyle. The strategies outlined above provide a roadmap for individuals seeking to foster balance, resilience, and a healthier response to stress in the midst of today's fast-paced world.

By incorporating these lifestyle strategies into daily routines, individuals can empower themselves to manage stress more effectively and support optimal cortisol regulation. The journey towards a balanced and harmonious relationship with stress involves not only adopting specific practices but also cultivating a mindset that prioritizes well-being, self-care, and the recognition of the body's innate ability to restore balance when provided with the right conditions.

Nutrition and Cortisol Balance

In the intricate dance of hormonal regulation, cortisol, often dubbed the "stress hormone," plays a central role. The interplay between nutrition and cortisol balance is a dynamic and essential aspect of maintaining overall health and well-being. This exploration delves into the impact of nutrition on cortisol levels, offering insights into how dietary choices influence the body's stress response and providing practical strategies for achieving a harmonious cortisol balance.

Understanding Cortisol and Its Role:

Cortisol, produced by the adrenal glands, is a steroid hormone that serves as a key player in the body's response to stress. In times of perceived threat or stress, cortisol is released as part of the "fight or flight" response, mobilizing energy stores and preparing the body for immediate action.

While this acute stress response is a crucial survival mechanism, chronic elevation of cortisol levels can lead to a range of health issues, including metabolic imbalances, immune suppression, and cognitive impairments.

The intricate relationship between nutrition and cortisol balance is rooted in the fact that dietary choices directly influence the body's hormonal milieu. Nutrients obtained from the diet play a role in supporting or challenging the stress response system, making nutrition a crucial factor in achieving and maintaining cortisol balance.

Nutrient-Rich Diet and Cortisol Regulation:

1. Balanced Macronutrients: A well-balanced intake of macronutrients—carbohydrates, proteins, and fats—is fundamental to cortisol regulation. Each macronutrient plays a unique role in supporting the body's energy needs and hormonal balance.

   - Carbohydrates: Complex carbohydrates, such as whole grains, fruits, and vegetables, provide a steady source of glucose, the primary fuel for the brain and body. Maintaining stable blood sugar levels is essential for preventing excessive cortisol release. Sudden drops in blood sugar, often associated with refined sugars and simple carbohydrates, can trigger a stress response and lead to elevated cortisol levels.

- Proteins: Adequate protein intake supports muscle health and provides amino acids necessary for various physiological processes, including the synthesis of hormones. Including lean protein sources, such as poultry, fish, tofu, and legumes, in the diet contributes to overall well-being and may help regulate cortisol levels.

- Fats: Healthy fats, particularly omega-3 fatty acids found in fatty fish, flaxseeds, and walnuts, are crucial for brain health and may have a protective effect against excessive cortisol release. Including sources of healthy fats in the diet supports a balanced hormonal response.

2. Micronutrients and Antioxidants: Micronutrients, including vitamins and minerals, play a vital role in supporting the body's stress response and cortisol balance. Antioxidants, in particular, help protect cells from oxidative stress, which is associated with chronic inflammation and cortisol dysregulation.

- Vitamin C: Found in citrus fruits, berries, and vegetables, vitamin C is an antioxidant that supports the immune system and may help modulate cortisol levels during times of stress.

- Vitamin B Complex: B-vitamins, including B6 and B12, are involved in the production and regulation of neurotransmitters and hormones, including cortisol. Sources of B-vitamins include whole grains, leafy greens, and lean meats.

- Magnesium: Magnesium is essential for numerous enzymatic reactions in the body, and adequate magnesium levels may help regulate cortisol. Magnesium-rich foods include leafy green vegetables, nuts, seeds, and whole grains.

- Zinc: Zinc is involved in immune function and may play a role in cortisol regulation. Foods rich in zinc include meat, dairy products, and nuts.

3. Hydration and Cortisol Dynamics: Proper hydration is a fundamental aspect of cortisol balance. Dehydration can lead to an increase in cortisol levels as the body perceives dehydration as a stressor. Maintaining adequate fluid intake supports overall health and helps the body manage stress more efficiently.

- Water: Staying well-hydrated by consuming an adequate amount of water throughout the day is essential for optimal physiological function. Decaffeinated herbal teas and infused water with slices of citrus fruits or cucumber are refreshing alternatives.

- Limiting Stimulants: Excessive caffeine intake, found in coffee, tea, and certain energy drinks, can contribute to dehydration and may trigger cortisol release. Moderation in caffeine consumption, particularly in the afternoon and evening, supports a balanced cortisol rhythm.

Nutritional Strategies for Cortisol Management:

1. Balancing Blood Sugar Levels:

   - Regular Meal Timing: Eating regular, balanced meals and snacks throughout the day helps maintain stable blood sugar levels. Skipping meals or relying on irregular eating patterns can contribute to fluctuations in blood sugar, triggering cortisol release.

   - Complex Carbohydrates: Emphasizing complex carbohydrates, such as whole grains, legumes, and vegetables, provides a sustained release of glucose and supports cortisol regulation.

   - Limiting Refined Sugars: Minimizing the intake of refined sugars and processed foods helps prevent spikes and crashes in blood sugar, which can activate the stress response.

2. Incorporating Adaptogenic Foods:

   - Adaptogens are a category of herbs and foods that may help the body adapt to stress and maintain balance. Examples include ashwagandha, rhodiola, and holy basil.

   - Green Tea: The polyphenols in green tea, particularly L-theanine, have calming effects and may help modulate cortisol levels. Opting for decaffeinated green tea in the evening can provide relaxation benefits without the stimulant effect.

3. Omega-3 Fatty Acids:

   - Including fatty fish (such as salmon, mackerel, and sardines), flaxseeds, chia seeds, and walnuts in the diet provides omega-3 fatty acids, which have anti-inflammatory properties and may support cortisol balance.

   - Omega-3 supplements, such as fish oil capsules, can be considered under the guidance of a healthcare professional for those who may have difficulty obtaining sufficient omega-3s through dietary sources.

4. Herbs and Spices:

   - Certain herbs and spices are believed to have stress-modulating effects and may contribute to cortisol balance.

   - Turmeric: The active compound in turmeric, curcumin, has anti-inflammatory properties and may help regulate cortisol levels.

   - Ginger: Ginger has antioxidant and anti-inflammatory properties and may contribute to overall well-being.

- Chamomile: Chamomile tea is known for its calming effects and may help promote relaxation.

5. Protein-Rich Snacks:

   - Including protein-rich snacks between meals can help stabilize blood sugar levels and prevent cortisol spikes.

   - Options such as Greek yogurt with nuts, hummus with carrot sticks, or a small serving of lean protein can provide a sustained source of energy.

Potential Pitfalls and Individual Variations:

While general nutritional guidelines can serve as a foundation for cortisol balance, it's essential to recognize that individual responses to dietary changes may vary. Additionally, certain medical conditions, medications, and individual health status can influence cortisol dynamics.

1. Dietary Restrictions:

   - Low-Carbohydrate Diets: Very low-carbohydrate diets may lead to increased cortisol levels, especially if not well-balanced with other macronutrients. It's important to prioritize complex carbohydrates and monitor individual responses to low-carb approaches.

   - Fasting and Intermittent Fasting: While intermittent fasting has gained popularity, prolonged fasting may activate the stress response and elevate cortisol levels. Individuals considering fasting approaches should do so under professional guidance and monitor their overall well-being.

2. Individual Variations:

   - Metabolic Variability: Individual metabolic variations can influence responses to certain foods. Monitoring energy levels, mood, and overall well-being can provide insights into how specific dietary choices affect cortisol dynamics.

   - Food Sensitivities: Undiagnosed food sensitivities or allergies can contribute to inflammation and stress in the body. Identifying and addressing such sensitivities may positively impact cortisol regulation.

Conclusion:

Navigating the intricate relationship between nutrition and cortisol balance requires a personalized and holistic approach. While certain dietary principles can serve as a foundation for stress management, individual variations, health conditions, and lifestyle factors must be considered.

By embracing a nutrient-rich, well-balanced diet, incorporating adaptogenic foods, and being mindful of lifestyle choices, individuals can contribute to a healthier cortisol balance. Additionally, staying attuned to the body's signals and seeking professional guidance when needed ensures a comprehensive and individualized approach to stress management through nutrition.

In the pursuit of holistic well-being, the synergy between nutrition and cortisol regulation offers a pathway to resilience, supporting the body's ability to adapt and thrive in the face of life's stressors.

Exercise for Cortisol Control

In the realm of stress management, exercise stands out as a powerful ally, offering not just physical benefits but also a profound impact on hormonal balance. Cortisol, the primary stress hormone, is intricately linked to the body's response to exercise. This exploration delves into the relationship between exercise and cortisol control, unveiling the mechanisms at play, the types of exercise that prove most effective, and practical strategies for harnessing the stress-relieving potential of physical activity.

Understanding Cortisol's Role in Stress and Exercise:

Cortisol, produced by the adrenal glands, is a central player in the body's stress response system. When faced with a stressor, whether physical or psychological, cortisol levels surge to mobilize energy reserves and prepare the body for action. While this acute stress response is crucial for

survival, chronic elevation of cortisol, often associated with persistent stress, can lead to a range of health issues, including immune suppression, metabolic imbalances, and cognitive impairments.

Exercise, as a form of physical stress, activates the same stress response system. However, the unique dynamics of exercise-induced cortisol release differ from the chronic elevation associated with ongoing stressors. Understanding the nuances of cortisol's role during exercise provides insights into how physical activity can be harnessed for stress management.

Types of Exercise and Cortisol Dynamics:

1. Aerobic Exercise:

   - Cardiovascular Benefits: Aerobic exercise, such as running, cycling, and swimming, is known for its cardiovascular benefits. During aerobic activity, cortisol levels typically increase in response to the physical stress, but they return to baseline relatively quickly after exercise cessation.

   - Moderate Intensity: Moderate-intensity aerobic exercise is often associated with optimal cortisol control. Engaging in activities like brisk walking or jogging for 30 to 60 minutes can promote a balanced cortisol response without inducing excessive stress.

   - Duration Matters: While short bursts of high-intensity aerobic exercise can trigger cortisol spikes, regular participation in longer duration, moderate-intensity aerobic sessions is generally well-tolerated and contributes to cortisol regulation.

2. Strength Training:

   - Muscle Building and Hormonal Response: Strength or resistance training, involving activities like weightlifting or bodyweight exercises, promotes muscle building and triggers a hormonal response, including the release of cortisol.

   - Short-Term Elevation: While cortisol levels may rise during a strength training session, the elevation is typically short-term and part of the natural hormonal response to exercise stress.

   - Hormonal Adaptations: Over time, the body may adapt to the stress of strength training, leading to improved cortisol regulation. Regular strength training sessions contribute to increased muscle mass, which can enhance the body's ability to manage cortisol.

3. High-Intensity Interval Training (HIIT):

   - Brief Intense Bursts: HIIT involves short bursts of intense exercise followed by periods of rest or lower-intensity activity. While HIIT can lead to acute increases in cortisol during the intense phases, it has been shown to support overall cortisol regulation when implemented as part of a well-rounded exercise routine.

- Time-Efficient: HIIT is praised for its time efficiency, making it an attractive option for individuals with busy schedules. The combination of intense effort and recovery periods appears to offer benefits for cortisol control.

- Individual Variations: HIIT may not be suitable for everyone, and individual responses to this form of exercise can vary. Consulting with a healthcare or fitness professional can help determine its appropriateness based on individual health and fitness levels.

Exercise-Induced Cortisol Regulation: The Mechanisms:

1. Endorphin Release:

- Natural Stress Relievers: Exercise triggers the release of endorphins, often referred to as "feel-good" hormones. The presence of endorphins helps counteract the potential stress response, contributing to an improved mood and reduced perception of stress.

- Endorphins and Cortisol: The release of endorphins during exercise is believed to interact with cortisol, influencing the overall stress response. Regular exercise contributes to the development of a more robust endorphin response, which may aid in cortisol regulation over time.

2. Hormonal Adaptations:

- Training the Stress Response: Regular, consistent exercise trains the body's stress response system. Over time, the body becomes more efficient at responding to stressors, leading to improved cortisol regulation.

- Cortisol Adaptations: The adaptation process involves the body becoming less reactive to the same level of stress. This phenomenon may contribute to a more controlled cortisol response during and after exercise.

3. Improvement in Sleep Quality:

- Reciprocal Relationship: Exercise has a reciprocal relationship with sleep—regular physical activity improves sleep quality, and quality sleep supports cortisol regulation.

- Sleep and Cortisol: Adequate, restorative sleep is crucial for cortisol balance. Exercise promotes better sleep, and the improved sleep quality contributes to a more balanced cortisol rhythm.

4. Psychological Benefits:

- Stress Reduction: Exercise has well-documented psychological benefits, including stress reduction. Engaging in physical activity provides a valuable outlet for stress, promoting mental well-being and influencing cortisol regulation.

- Cognitive Benefits: Regular exercise is associated with improved cognitive function and resilience to stress. These cognitive benefits may contribute to a more adaptive cortisol response.

Strategies for Harnessing Exercise for Cortisol Control:

1. Consistency is Key:

- Establishing a Routine: Consistent, regular exercise is essential for long-term cortisol regulation. Establishing a routine that includes both aerobic and strength training components provides comprehensive benefits for hormonal balance.

- Frequency and Duration: Aim for at least 150 minutes of moderate-intensity aerobic exercise per week, along with strength training activities at least two days per week. Adjust the frequency and duration based on individual fitness levels and goals.

2. Variety in Exercise Modalities:

- Cross-Training: Incorporating a variety of exercise modalities, including aerobic, strength training, and flexibility exercises, offers diverse benefits for overall health and cortisol regulation.

- Enjoyable Activities: Choosing activities that are enjoyable increases the likelihood of consistency. Whether it's dancing, hiking, or playing a sport, finding pleasure in physical activity contributes to a positive stress-management experience.

3. Mindful Movement Practices:

- Yoga and Tai Chi: Mindful movement practices, such as yoga and tai chi, combine physical activity with mental focus and breath awareness. These practices have been associated with improved cortisol regulation and stress reduction.

- Mind-Body Connection: The mind-body connection cultivated in practices like yoga may enhance the body's ability to respond to stressors more adaptively, influencing cortisol release.

4. Individualized Approach:

- Listen to the Body: Paying attention to individual responses to exercise is crucial. While some individuals may thrive on high-intensity workouts, others may find gentler forms of exercise more suitable for their stress management needs.

- Consult with Professionals: Consulting with fitness professionals or healthcare providers can help tailor an exercise program to individual health status, fitness levels, and stress management goals.

5. Post-Exercise Recovery:

- Importance of Recovery: Incorporating adequate recovery time is crucial for overall well-being and cortisol control. Balancing challenging workouts with rest days or lower-intensity activities prevents overtraining and excessive cortisol release.

- Sleep Hygiene: Recognizing the synergy between exercise and sleep, prioritizing good sleep hygiene practices further supports cortisol regulation. This includes maintaining a consistent sleep schedule, creating a conducive sleep environment, and minimizing stimulants before bedtime.

Potential Pitfalls and Considerations:

1. Overtraining:

- Balancing Intensity: Overtraining, characterized by excessive exercise without adequate recovery, can lead to elevated cortisol levels. Balancing the intensity and duration of workouts is crucial for preventing overtraining.

- Individual Tolerance: Individual tolerance to exercise varies, and it's essential to recognize signs of fatigue, burnout, or persistent soreness. Adjusting the exercise routine based on individual responses promotes sustainable cortisol control.

2. Chronic Stress and Cortisol Dysregulation:

- Underlying Health Conditions: Chronic stress, whether related to personal, work, or health factors, can contribute to cortisol dysregulation. Individuals facing chronic stress should consider comprehensive stress management strategies, including exercise, in consultation with healthcare professionals.

- Addressing Underlying Stressors: While exercise is a valuable tool for stress management, addressing the underlying causes of chronic stress is crucial. Seeking support from mental health professionals, adopting stress-reduction techniques, and making lifestyle adjustments contribute to a holistic approach.

Conclusion:

Exercise, with its multifaceted benefits, emerges as a formidable tool in the quest for cortisol control and stress management. From the release of endorphins to hormonal adaptations and improvements in sleep quality, the impact of exercise on cortisol regulation extends beyond the physical realm.

Individuals seeking to harness the stress-relieving potential of exercise should embrace a holistic approach, incorporating a variety of activities, recognizing individual preferences and tolerances, and prioritizing post-exercise recovery. With consistency, mindfulness, and a personalized approach, exercise becomes a potent ally in the journey toward cortisol control, fostering not just physical fitness but also mental resilience and overall well-being.

Sleep's Crucial Role in Cortisol Management

In the intricate symphony of hormonal balance, sleep emerges as a conductor, orchestrating the ebb and flow of cortisol—the primary stress hormone. The relationship between sleep and cortisol management is profound, with sleep quality and duration playing pivotal roles in determining the body's ability to regulate stress effectively. This exploration delves into the intricate connections between sleep and cortisol, unveiling the mechanisms at play, the consequences of sleep disruption on cortisol dynamics, and practical strategies for cultivating a harmonious relationship between sleep and stress management.

Understanding Cortisol and Its Circadian Rhythm:

Cortisol, produced by the adrenal glands, is a steroid hormone that plays a multifaceted role in the body. While often associated with the stress response, cortisol is involved in various physiological processes, including metabolism, immune function, and the sleep-wake cycle. The secretion of cortisol follows a circadian rhythm, peaking in the early morning to promote wakefulness and gradually declining throughout the day, reaching its lowest levels in the late evening and early night.

The intricate dance of cortisol's circadian rhythm is closely intertwined with the body's internal clock, the circadian system. This system, regulated by the suprachiasmatic nucleus in the brain, synchronizes various physiological processes with the natural light-dark cycle. Disruptions to this circadian rhythm, such as those caused by irregular sleep patterns or insufficient sleep, can impact cortisol dynamics, leading to dysregulation and potential health consequences.

The Impact of Sleep on Cortisol Dynamics:

1. Quality and Duration:

- Balancing Act: Adequate, high-quality sleep is essential for maintaining a balanced cortisol rhythm. The duration and depth of sleep directly influence the body's ability to regulate cortisol effectively.

- Deep Sleep and Cortisol Suppression: During deep sleep, cortisol levels typically experience a significant drop. This suppression of cortisol during deep sleep allows the body to recover and regenerate, promoting overall well-being.

- Role of REM Sleep: Rapid Eye Movement (REM) sleep, another crucial stage of the sleep cycle, is associated with vivid dreaming and plays a role in emotional processing. While cortisol levels may rise slightly during REM sleep, the overall pattern supports cortisol regulation.

2. Circadian Rhythm Synchronization:

- Alignment with Natural Light-Dark Cycle: The circadian rhythm of cortisol is intricately connected to the natural light-dark cycle. Exposure to natural light in the morning helps synchronize the circadian system, promoting a healthy cortisol peak in the early waking hours.

- Melatonin and Cortisol Relationship: Melatonin, the hormone responsible for promoting sleep, exhibits an inverse relationship with cortisol. As melatonin levels rise in the evening, cortisol levels decline, signaling the body's transition into restful sleep.

- Shift Work and Cortisol Disruption: Disruptions to the circadian rhythm, such as those experienced by individuals working night shifts or irregular hours, can lead to cortisol dysregulation. The body may struggle to adapt to a shifted sleep-wake cycle, impacting overall cortisol dynamics.

3. Sleep Architecture and Cortisol Fluctuations:

- Sleep Stages and Hormonal Regulation: The various sleep stages, including non-REM and REM sleep, contribute to hormonal regulation. Disturbances in sleep architecture, such as fragmented sleep or frequent awakenings, can disrupt the finely tuned balance of cortisol release.

- Cortisol Awakening Response (CAR): The cortisol awakening response (CAR) is a natural surge in cortisol levels that occurs within the first hour of waking. This response is influenced by factors such as anticipation of the day ahead and is typically blunted in individuals with sleep disturbances or irregular sleep patterns.

Consequences of Sleep Disruption on Cortisol Regulation:

1. Elevated Cortisol Levels:

- Chronic Sleep Deprivation: Prolonged sleep deprivation or chronic insufficient sleep is associated with elevated cortisol levels. The body perceives sleep deprivation as a stressor, leading to an overactive stress response and sustained cortisol release.

- Stress and Cortisol Dysregulation: The bidirectional relationship between stress and cortisol can create a cycle where heightened stress contributes to sleep disruption, and inadequate sleep, in turn, exacerbates stress and cortisol dysregulation.

2. Metabolic Impacts:

- Insulin Sensitivity: Disrupted cortisol levels due to insufficient sleep may impact insulin sensitivity, potentially contributing to metabolic issues and an increased risk of type 2 diabetes.

- Appetite Regulation: Cortisol influences appetite regulation, and sleep disruption can lead to changes in hunger hormones, potentially contributing to overeating and weight gain.

3. Immune Function:

- Immunosuppression: Adequate sleep is crucial for maintaining a robust immune system. Chronic elevation of cortisol, resulting from sleep disruption, may contribute to immunosuppression, increasing susceptibility to infections and illnesses.

- Inflammatory Response: Cortisol has anti-inflammatory properties, and disruptions to cortisol rhythms can contribute to an overactive inflammatory response. Chronic inflammation is associated with various health conditions, including cardiovascular disease and autoimmune disorders.

4. Cognitive Function:

- Memory and Learning: Sleep plays a vital role in memory consolidation and learning. Cortisol, as a modulator of cognitive function, is influenced by the restorative effects of sleep. Sleep disruption may impair these cognitive processes, affecting memory and learning abilities.

- Emotional Regulation: Cortisol is involved in emotional regulation, and sleep disturbances can impact mood and stress resilience. Chronic sleep deprivation may contribute to heightened emotional reactivity and increased vulnerability to stressors.

Strategies for Cultivating Healthy Sleep and Cortisol Regulation:

1. Establishing a Consistent Sleep Schedule:

- Prioritizing Regularity: Going to bed and waking up at the same time each day helps synchronize the circadian rhythm and promotes a consistent cortisol pattern.

- Weekend Adjustments: While some flexibility is acceptable, minimizing drastic changes in sleep schedules, even on weekends, contributes to overall circadian rhythm stability.

2. Creating a Sleep-Conducive Environment:

- Optimizing Sleep Environment: Designing a bedroom conducive to sleep involves factors such as comfortable bedding, adequate room darkness, and maintaining a cool, quiet, and clutter-free space.

- Limiting Screen Time: Exposure to electronic devices emitting blue light before bedtime can disrupt melatonin production. Establishing a screen-free period before sleep supports the natural transition to restful sleep.

3. Managing Stress and Relaxation Techniques:

- Mindfulness Practices: Incorporating mindfulness techniques, such as deep breathing, progressive muscle relaxation, or meditation, can help reduce stress and promote relaxation.

- Stress Reduction Activities: Engaging in activities that promote relaxation, such as reading, gentle stretching, or taking a warm bath before bedtime, signals to the body that it's time to unwind.

4. Limiting Stimulants:

- Caffeine and Nicotine: Limiting the consumption of stimulants, such as caffeine and nicotine, particularly in the hours leading up to bedtime, supports a smoother transition to sleep.

- Alcohol Moderation: While alcohol may initially induce drowsiness, excessive consumption can disrupt sleep cycles and contribute to cortisol dysregulation. Moderation is key.

5. Regular Physical Activity:

- Exercise and Sleep: Regular physical activity, especially aerobic exercise, contributes to better sleep quality and supports cortisol regulation. However, intense exercise close to bedtime may have stimulating effects, so it's advisable to complete workouts several hours before sleep.

- Outdoor Activity: Exposure to natural light, especially in the morning, helps regulate circadian rhythms. Incorporating outdoor activities into the daily routine contributes to a healthy sleep-wake cycle.

6. Balanced Nutrition:

- Meal Timing: Avoiding heavy meals close to bedtime and opting for a balanced evening snack can support stable blood sugar levels and contribute to a more restful sleep.

- Hydration: Maintaining adequate hydration is essential, but excessive fluid intake before bedtime may lead to disruptions in sleep due to nighttime bathroom visits.

7. Professional Guidance:

- Consulting Sleep Professionals: Individuals experiencing persistent sleep difficulties or disruptions that significantly impact daily functioning should consider seeking guidance from sleep specialists or healthcare professionals.

- Sleep Studies: In cases of chronic sleep disorders, such as sleep apnea or insomnia, diagnostic sleep studies may provide valuable insights into underlying issues and inform targeted interventions.

Conclusion:

The intricate interplay between sleep and cortisol is a testament to the body's finely tuned mechanisms for maintaining balance and well-being. Recognizing the pivotal role of sleep in cortisol regulation underscores the importance of cultivating healthy sleep habits as a cornerstone of stress management.

By prioritizing consistent sleep schedules, creating a sleep-conducive environment, managing stress through relaxation techniques, and adopting a balanced lifestyle, individuals can nurture the

delicate dance between sleep and cortisol. As the body's internal conductor, orchestrating the rhythm of hormonal harmony, quality sleep emerges not only as a remedy for fatigue but as a profound contributor to overall health, resilience, and the body's ability to navigate the challenges of daily life with grace.

Chapter Four
Stress Reduction Techniques

In the fast-paced and demanding landscape of modern life, stress has become a ubiquitous companion for many. However, the detrimental effects of chronic stress on physical and mental well-being underscore the importance of adopting effective stress reduction techniques. This exploration delves into a variety of strategies aimed at mitigating stress, promoting resilience, and fostering a sense of balance in the midst of life's challenges. From mindfulness practices to physical activity and creative outlets, the array of techniques available provides a versatile toolkit for individuals seeking to navigate the complexities of daily life with greater ease.

1. Mindfulness and Meditation: Cultivating Presence in the Moment

Mindfulness and meditation are ancient practices that have found renewed relevance in the contemporary quest for stress reduction. These techniques center around cultivating a focused awareness of the present moment, allowing individuals to observe their thoughts and feelings without judgment. The benefits extend beyond the practice itself, influencing how individuals respond to stressors in their daily lives.

- Mindfulness Meditation: Mindfulness meditation involves paying deliberate attention to the present moment. This can be achieved through techniques such as focused breathing, body scans, or guided imagery. Regular practice enhances the ability to stay present, fostering a calmer response to stressors.

- Mindful Breathing: Taking slow, intentional breaths and focusing on the sensation of each inhalation and exhalation can anchor the mind in the present moment, reducing anxiety and promoting relaxation.

- Body Scan Meditation: This practice involves directing attention to different parts of the body, noticing sensations without judgment. It promotes relaxation and body awareness, helping individuals release tension.

- Transcendental Meditation: Transcendental Meditation (TM) is a specific form of mantra meditation that involves silently repeating a mantra for 15-20 minutes, twice daily. Proponents suggest that this practice can lead to a deep state of restful awareness, reducing stress and promoting overall well-being.

- Mantra Repetition: The repetition of a mantra during TM is thought to facilitate a state of restful alertness, promoting relaxation and reducing the impact of stress on the mind and body.

2. Physical Activity: Energizing the Body and Mind

Regular physical activity is a powerful antidote to stress, offering benefits for both the body and mind. Exercise has been shown to reduce cortisol levels, improve mood, and enhance overall resilience to stressors.

- Aerobic Exercise: Aerobic exercise, such as walking, running, cycling, or swimming, is known for its mood-enhancing effects. The release of endorphins, often referred to as "feel-good" hormones, contributes to a sense of well-being and reduces the perception of stress.

- Nature Walks: Combining the benefits of aerobic exercise with exposure to nature amplifies the stress-reducing effects. Nature walks or outdoor activities provide a double dose of well-being.

- Yoga: Yoga is a holistic practice that integrates physical postures, breath control, and meditation. It emphasizes the mind-body connection, making it an effective stress reduction technique.

- Gentle Yoga: Practices such as Hatha or restorative yoga focus on gentle movements and breath awareness. These forms of yoga are accessible to individuals of varying fitness levels and can be particularly effective for stress reduction.

- High-Intensity Interval Training (HIIT): HIIT involves short bursts of intense exercise followed by rest or lower-intensity periods. While it is vigorous, the time-efficient nature of HIIT makes it an attractive option for those with busy schedules.

   - Quick Workouts: HIIT workouts can be completed in a relatively short time, making them suitable for individuals with time constraints. The intensity of these workouts can enhance mood and reduce stress.

3. Creative Outlets: Expressing Emotions Through Art

Engaging in creative activities provides an outlet for self-expression and emotional release. Whether through visual arts, writing, or music, the act of creating can be a therapeutic and fulfilling way to manage stress.

- Art Therapy: Art therapy involves using visual arts as a form of expression and self-exploration. It can be particularly beneficial for individuals who find it challenging to articulate their emotions verbally.

   - Drawing and Painting: The act of drawing or painting allows individuals to externalize their thoughts and emotions, providing a tangible representation of their internal experiences.

- Journaling: Journaling is a reflective practice that involves writing about thoughts, feelings, and experiences. It serves as a cathartic outlet for processing emotions and gaining insights into stressors.

   - Gratitude Journal: Focusing on positive aspects by maintaining a gratitude journal can shift the perspective, fostering a sense of appreciation and reducing the impact of stressors.

- Music and Relaxation: Listening to or creating music has profound effects on emotions and stress levels. Music therapy is utilized to promote relaxation and emotional expression.

   - Playing an Instrument: Learning to play a musical instrument provides a creative and absorbing activity. The process of creating music can be a meditative and stress-relieving experience.

4. Breathing Techniques: Harnessing the Power of Breath

Conscious control of breath is a simple yet potent stress reduction technique. Breathwork practices help regulate the autonomic nervous system, promoting a shift from the stress response to a more relaxed state.

- Deep Breathing: Deep breathing involves taking slow, deliberate breaths, focusing on expanding the diaphragm. This practice activates the body's relaxation response, reducing tension and promoting a sense of calm.

- Diaphragmatic Breathing: Also known as abdominal or belly breathing, this technique involves breathing deeply into the diaphragm rather than shallow chest breathing. It can be practiced in various positions, including sitting or lying down.

- Box Breathing: Box breathing, also known as square breathing, involves inhaling, holding the breath, exhaling, and holding the breath again, each for an equal duration. This rhythmic pattern helps regulate the breath and induces a state of relaxation.

- 4-4-4-4 Pattern: Inhale for a count of four, hold for four counts, exhale for four counts, and hold the breath again for four counts. This cycle can be repeated several times.

5. Time Management: Organizing and Prioritizing Responsibilities

Effective time management is a practical approach to stress reduction, allowing individuals to organize their tasks, set priorities, and create a sense of control over their responsibilities.

- Prioritization: Identifying and prioritizing tasks based on importance and deadlines prevents feeling overwhelmed. Breaking larger tasks into smaller, manageable steps makes the workload more achievable.

- Eisenhower Matrix: Categorizing tasks into urgent-important, not urgent-important, urgent-not important, and not urgent-not important can guide effective prioritization.

- Goal Setting: Establishing clear and realistic goals provides a roadmap for success. Setting achievable milestones and celebrating accomplishments along the way fosters a sense of progress.

- SMART Goals: Goals should be Specific, Measurable, Achievable, Relevant, and Time-bound. This framework enhances clarity and increases the likelihood of successful goal attainment.

- Effective Planning: Planning involves creating a roadmap for daily, weekly, or monthly activities. Using tools such as planners, calendars, or digital apps can help individuals stay organized and reduce the stress associated with forgetfulness or last-minute tasks.

- Time Blocking: Allocating specific time blocks for different tasks helps create structure and prevents the feeling of being constantly rushed or overwhelmed.

6. Social Connection: Building Supportive Relationships

Social connections play a crucial role in emotional well-being and stress resilience. Nurturing positive relationships and seeking support from others can alleviate the emotional burden of stress.

- Communication: Open and honest communication fosters understanding and connection. Sharing thoughts and feelings with trusted friends, family members, or colleagues can provide emotional support and perspective.

- Active Listening: Actively listening to others and feeling heard is a fundamental aspect of supportive communication. Practicing empathy and validation strengthens social bonds.

- Social Activities: Engaging in social activities and spending time with loved ones provides a sense of belonging and emotional support. Positive social interactions contribute to a buffer against stress.

- Shared Hobbies: Participating in activities or hobbies with others fosters a sense of community and shared enjoyment, promoting positive social connections.

7. Relaxation Techniques: Unwinding for Overall Well-being

Intentional relaxation techniques offer a direct counterbalance to the physiological and psychological effects of stress. Incorporating practices that induce a state of relaxation contributes to overall well-being.

- Progressive Muscle Relaxation (PMR): PMR involves systematically tensing and then relaxing different muscle groups. This technique helps release physical tension and promotes a sense of relaxation throughout the body.

- Body Scan: A variation of PMR, the body scan involves mentally focusing on each part of the body, progressively releasing tension and promoting a state of calm.

- Hot Baths or Showers: Immersing oneself in a warm bath or taking a hot shower can be soothing for both the body and mind. The warmth helps relax muscles, and the sensory experience provides a calming effect.

- Aromatherapy: Adding calming scents, such as lavender or chamomile, to the bath or using essential oils in a diffuser enhances the relaxation experience.

- Nature Exposure: Spending time in natural settings has been shown to have stress-reducing effects. Whether through outdoor walks, hikes, or simply sitting in a park, connecting with nature promotes a sense of tranquility.

- Forest Bathing: Forest bathing, or shinrin-yoku, is a Japanese practice involving immersing oneself in a forest environment. This practice has been associated with reduced stress and improved well-being.

Conclusion: Crafting a Personalized Approach to Stress Reduction

The diversity of stress reduction techniques reflects the individualized nature of stress management. Crafting a personalized approach involves exploring different strategies, observing their effects, and tailoring practices to align with individual preferences and needs.

Whether through the stillness of meditation, the invigoration of physical activity, the catharsis of creative expression, or the intentional cultivation of social connections, individuals have a wealth of options to choose from. By integrating a variety of stress reduction techniques into daily life, individuals can build resilience, enhance overall well-being, and navigate the complexities of modern existence with a greater sense of ease and balance.

Mindfulness and Cortisol: A Synergistic Approach

In the intricate dance between mind and body, the relationship between mindfulness and cortisol emerges as a powerful and nuanced interplay. Mindfulness, rooted in ancient contemplative traditions, involves cultivating a heightened awareness of the present moment without judgment. Cortisol, the primary stress hormone, responds to the body's perceived threats and challenges. This exploration delves into the profound synergy between mindfulness practices and cortisol regulation, unraveling the mechanisms at play and highlighting the transformative impact of this harmonious relationship on stress reduction and overall well-being.

Understanding Mindfulness: The Art of Present-Moment Awareness

Mindfulness, often encapsulated in practices such as meditation and mindful breathing, is grounded in the concept of bringing full attention to the present moment. Developed through traditions like Buddhism, mindfulness has transcended its cultural origins to become a widely embraced approach to mental well-being in contemporary contexts.

1. Mindful Meditation:

   - Breath Awareness: Mindful meditation frequently centers around the breath, with practitioners focusing on the inhalation and exhalation. This simple yet profound practice cultivates a non-judgmental awareness of the breath, anchoring the mind in the present moment.

- Observing Thoughts: Mindfulness encourages the observation of thoughts without attachment or judgment. Practitioners learn to witness the ebb and flow of thoughts, fostering a detached awareness that diminishes the emotional charge often associated with stressors.

2. Body Scan:

- Tuning into Sensations: The body scan is a mindfulness technique involving a systematic focus on different parts of the body. Practitioners mentally scan through each area, noting sensations without judgment. This practice enhances body awareness and promotes relaxation.

- Tension Release: By acknowledging and releasing physical tension, the body scan contributes to a sense of ease and calm. This physical relaxation complements the mental aspects of mindfulness, creating a holistic stress-reducing effect.

3. Mindful Movement Practices:

- Yoga and Tai Chi: Mindful movement practices combine physical activity with intentional breath awareness and mental focus. Yoga, with its diverse postures and flows, and Tai Chi, known for its slow and deliberate movements, exemplify these embodied mindfulness practices.

- Embodied Presence: Engaging in mindful movement fosters a connection between the mind and body. This integrated approach contributes to stress reduction by promoting physical well-being and mental clarity.

Cortisol and the Stress Response: Navigating Life's Challenges

Cortisol, produced by the adrenal glands, is a central player in the body's stress response system. When confronted with a perceived threat or challenge, the brain signals the release of cortisol, mobilizing energy reserves and preparing the body for action. While this acute stress response is crucial for survival, chronic elevation of cortisol due to persistent stress can lead to a range of health issues.

1. Cortisol's Role in the Body:

- Energy Mobilization: Cortisol plays a key role in mobilizing energy stores, particularly glucose, to fuel the body's response to stress. This prepares the individual to face challenges by providing the necessary resources for physical and mental exertion.

- Immunosuppressive Effects: Chronic elevation of cortisol can suppress the immune system, making individuals more susceptible to infections and illnesses. Balancing cortisol levels is essential for maintaining a robust immune response.

2. The Stress Response System:

- Hypothalamus-Pituitary-Adrenal (HPA) Axis: The HPA axis is a complex system involving the hypothalamus, pituitary gland, and adrenal glands. When the brain perceives a stressor, the HPA axis is activated, leading to the release of cortisol.

- Feedback Mechanism: Cortisol exerts negative feedback on the HPA axis, signaling the system to downregulate cortisol production once the stressor has passed. Chronic stress can disrupt this feedback loop, contributing to sustained cortisol elevation.

Mindfulness and Cortisol Regulation: A Synergetic Dance

The synergy between mindfulness practices and cortisol regulation lies in the ability of mindfulness to modulate the stress response. By fostering a state of present-moment awareness and altering the perception of stressors, mindfulness contributes to a more adaptive cortisol release pattern.

1. Reducing Psychological Stress:

   - Perception Shift: Mindfulness encourages individuals to observe their thoughts and emotions without getting entangled in them. This shift in perception allows for a more objective and non-reactive response to stressors, reducing the psychological impact.

   - Mindful Coping: Mindfulness equips individuals with tools to cope with stressors in a measured and intentional way. Rather than reacting impulsively, individuals learn to respond mindfully, mitigating the emotional toll on the body and, subsequently, cortisol levels.

2. Enhancing Emotional Regulation:

   - Embracing Emotional Resilience: Mindfulness fosters emotional resilience by creating a space between stimuli and response. This space allows individuals to choose their reactions consciously, preventing emotional reactivity that could contribute to cortisol elevation.

   - Mindful Acceptance: Rather than suppressing or avoiding challenging emotions, mindfulness encourages acceptance. This acknowledgment of emotions reduces internal conflict and the associated stress, positively influencing cortisol dynamics.

3. Body-Mind Connection:

   - Embodied Mindfulness: Mindfulness practices often emphasize the connection between the mind and body. By cultivating awareness of bodily sensations, practitioners develop a heightened sensitivity to stress-related tension, facilitating targeted relaxation.

   - Relaxation Response: Mindfulness triggers the relaxation response, a physiological state characterized by decreased heart rate, relaxed muscles, and improved mood. This counteracts the physiological manifestations of stress, including cortisol release.

Neuroplasticity and Cortical Changes:

The practice of mindfulness has been associated with structural changes in the brain, particularly in areas involved in stress regulation and emotional processing. These changes, driven by neuroplasticity, contribute to a more adaptive stress response.

1. Amygdala Modulation:

   - Reduced Amygdala Reactivity: The amygdala, a key player in the brain's emotional processing, is involved in initiating the stress response. Mindfulness practices have been linked to reduced amygdala reactivity, indicating a more measured response to stressors.

   - Emotional Regulation: By modulating the amygdala, mindfulness supports emotional regulation. This modulation may contribute to a dampened stress response, ultimately influencing cortisol release patterns.

2. Prefrontal Cortex Activation:

   - Enhanced Prefrontal Cortex Function: Mindfulness has been associated with increased activity in the prefrontal cortex, particularly in areas related to executive functions and self-regulation. This enhanced function contributes to better stress management.

   - Cognitive Control: The prefrontal cortex plays a role in cognitive control, allowing individuals to regulate emotions and responses to stress. Mindfulness practices strengthen these cognitive functions, influencing cortisol regulation.

Mindfulness-Based Interventions: Clinical Applications and Evidence

The integration of mindfulness into clinical interventions has gained traction in fields such as psychology and healthcare. Mindfulness-based interventions (MBIs) leverage mindfulness practices to address various conditions, including stress-related disorders, anxiety, and depression.

1. Mindfulness-Based Stress Reduction (MBSR):

   - Holistic Approach: MBSR, developed by Dr. Jon Kabat-Zinn, is a structured program that integrates mindfulness meditation and awareness practices. It is designed to enhance participants' ability to cope with stress and improve overall well-being.

   - Cortisol Reduction: Research indicates that MBSR is associated with reduced cortisol levels in individuals facing chronic stress. This suggests that the cultivation of mindfulness can have tangible effects on the body's stress hormone dynamics.

2. Mindfulness-Based Cognitive Therapy (MBCT):

- Combining Mindfulness with Cognitive Therapy: MBCT combines mindfulness practices with elements of cognitive therapy to prevent the recurrence of depression. It targets the interplay between negative thought patterns and emotional well-being.

- Preventing Cortisol Dysregulation: Studies suggest that MBCT may contribute to preventing cortisol dysregulation associated with depressive relapse. By addressing cognitive patterns and fostering mindfulness, the intervention influences stress response mechanisms.

Practical Applications of Mindfulness for Cortisol Regulation:

1. Daily Mindfulness Practice:

- Consistency is Key: Establishing a daily mindfulness practice, even if brief, fosters a cumulative impact on stress resilience. Consistency in practice reinforces the neural pathways associated with mindfulness and contributes to long-term cortisol regulation.

- Integration into Routine: Incorporating mindfulness into daily routines, such as mindful breathing during breaks or a short meditation before bedtime, promotes accessibility and sustainable practice.

2. Mindful Movement and Cortisol:

- Yoga for Stress Reduction: Mindful movement practices like yoga offer a dual benefit by combining physical activity with intentional breath awareness. Regular participation in yoga has been associated with reduced cortisol levels.

- Tai Chi for Cortisol Harmony: The slow and deliberate movements of Tai Chi, coupled with mindful breath control, create a conducive environment for cortisol regulation. Incorporating Tai Chi into a routine provides a mindful avenue for physical activity.

3. Mindfulness in Stressful Situations:

- Mindful Responses to Stressors: Applying mindfulness techniques in real-time during stressful situations enhances the ability to respond thoughtfully. Mindful breathing or a moment of present-moment awareness can interrupt the automatic stress response.

- Cultivating Mindful Habits: Establishing habits that prompt mindfulness during daily stressors, such as taking a few conscious breaths before responding to an email, builds a foundation for sustainable stress reduction.

Conclusion: The Transformative Alchemy of Mindfulness and Cortisol

In the symphony of stress and well-being, mindfulness and cortisol engage in a transformative dance. The deliberate cultivation of mindfulness offers individuals a profound tool to navigate the complexities of life with grace and resilience. By fostering present-moment awareness, altering perceptions of stressors, and influencing the brain's stress response circuitry, mindfulness acts as a harmonizing force.

The synergy between mindfulness and cortisol regulation extends beyond theoretical frameworks, finding empirical support in clinical interventions and scientific studies. Mindfulness-based programs demonstrate tangible effects on cortisol levels, offering a promising avenue for addressing stress-related conditions.

As individuals embark on their mindfulness journey, the alchemy between awareness and cortisol becomes not just a theoretical concept but a lived experience. Mindfulness becomes a companion in the quest for balance, providing a sanctuary of calm amidst life's storms. In this union, the individual discovers the power to not only manage stress but to transform the very fabric of their relationship with the inevitable challenges of existence.

Chapter Five

Real-life Examples of Cortisol Management Success

The journey towards effective cortisol management is a deeply personal one, often marked by unique challenges, resilience, and triumphs. Real-life examples serve as powerful narratives that illuminate the diverse paths individuals take in their quest for well-being. These stories not only offer inspiration but also provide practical insights into the strategies and habits that have proven successful in managing cortisol levels. In this exploration, we delve into real-life examples that showcase the triumphs of individuals who have navigated the complexities of stress, highlighting the varied approaches and lessons learned along the way.

1. Sarah's Mindful Living Transformation:

Sarah's journey towards cortisol management was marked by a profound shift in lifestyle and mindset. A high-powered executive, Sarah found herself entangled in a web of constant deadlines, late-night emails, and a relentless pursuit of professional success. The toll on her well-being was evident in disrupted sleep patterns, heightened anxiety, and a persistent feeling of burnout.

Strategies:

- Mindful Morning Rituals: Sarah recognized the importance of setting a positive tone for the day. She incorporated mindful morning rituals such as meditation and mindful breathing into her routine. Starting the day with intentional practices allowed her to manage stress more effectively.

- Work-Life Boundaries: Establishing clear boundaries between work and personal life became a priority. Sarah implemented practices such as turning off work-related notifications after a certain hour and creating dedicated spaces for relaxation at home.

- Regular Nature Walks: Sarah discovered the calming effects of nature. Regular walks in a nearby park became a cornerstone of her cortisol management strategy. The combination of physical activity and connection with nature provided a respite from the demands of her professional life.

Lessons Learned:

Sarah's story illustrates the transformative power of mindfulness and intentional living. By incorporating practices that prioritize well-being, she not only managed her cortisol levels but also experienced a profound shift in her overall quality of life.

2. Mike's Fitness Journey: From Stress to Strength:

Mike's cortisol management journey took a fitness-centric approach. A fitness enthusiast from a young age, Mike faced a period of heightened stress due to work pressures and personal challenges. Recognizing the impact on his mental and physical well-being, he decided to leverage his passion for fitness to counteract the effects of stress.

Strategies:

- Structured Exercise Routine: Mike developed a structured exercise routine that included a mix of cardiovascular exercises, strength training, and flexibility work. The routine not only served as a physical outlet but also became a time for mental rejuvenation.

- Mindful Nutrition: Understanding the connection between nutrition and cortisol, Mike made mindful choices in his diet. He focused on balanced meals with an emphasis on whole foods, ensuring he provided his body with the nutrients needed to manage stress effectively.

- Social Support Through Fitness: Mike found a supportive community through fitness classes and workout groups. The social connection and shared goals provided an additional layer of support, reducing the feelings of isolation that often accompany stress.

Lessons Learned:

Mike's journey showcases the symbiotic relationship between physical fitness and cortisol management. By channeling his passion for exercise into a structured routine, he not only improved his physical health but also cultivated a resilient mindset.

3. Emily's Holistic Healing:

Emily's cortisol management journey was rooted in holistic healing modalities. Facing a combination of work-related stress and personal challenges, Emily sought a comprehensive approach that addressed both the mind and body.

Strategies:

- Yoga and Mind-Body Practices: Emily embraced yoga and other mind-body practices as central components of her routine. The combination of physical postures, breathwork, and meditation provided a holistic approach to stress reduction.

- Therapeutic Support: Recognizing the importance of mental health, Emily sought therapeutic support. Regular counseling sessions allowed her to explore and address the underlying causes of stress, contributing to a more sustainable cortisol management strategy.

- Herbal Supplements: Emily incorporated herbal supplements known for their calming properties. Under the guidance of a healthcare professional, she explored natural options such as adaptogens and herbal teas to support her body's stress response.

Lessons Learned:

Emily's journey highlights the significance of a holistic approach to cortisol management. By addressing the interconnectedness of mind and body through practices like yoga and therapeutic support, she cultivated a resilient foundation for well-being.

4. James' Tech Detox for Stress Reduction:

James, a technology professional, realized the impact of constant connectivity on his stress levels. The incessant flow of emails, notifications, and screen time contributed to heightened cortisol levels and a sense of perpetual stress.

Strategies:

- Digital Detox Weekends: James implemented regular digital detox weekends where he consciously disconnected from screens and technology. This intentional break allowed his mind to reset and reduced the constant stimuli that contributed to stress.

- Establishing Tech-Free Zones: Recognizing the need for ongoing boundaries, James designated specific areas in his home as tech-free zones. This included keeping electronic devices out of the bedroom to create a conducive environment for restful sleep.

- Mindful Tech Consumption: James became more mindful of his technology consumption during work hours. Implementing practices such as the Pomodoro Technique, which involves structured work and break intervals, helped him maintain focus without succumbing to digital overwhelm.

Lessons Learned:

James' journey emphasizes the importance of establishing boundaries with technology for cortisol management. By intentionally creating spaces and times free from digital distractions, he regained a sense of control over his stress levels.

5. Maria's Journey to Boundaries and Balance:

Maria, a working mother, faced the challenge of balancing career responsibilities with family life. The constant juggling act took a toll on her stress levels, prompting her to reevaluate her priorities and implement strategies for better cortisol management.

Strategies:

- Work-Life Integration: Maria shifted her mindset from the concept of work-life balance to work-life integration. This involved identifying moments of synergy between work and family life, allowing her to seamlessly transition between roles without the stress of compartmentalization.

- Delegating Responsibilities: Recognizing the importance of support, Maria delegated responsibilities at work and at home. This included enlisting the help of family members and colleagues to share the load, reducing the pressure on her to handle everything alone.

- Mindful Time Management: Maria adopted mindful time management techniques, including setting realistic goals and priorities. This approach allowed her to focus on what truly mattered, minimizing the stress associated with an overwhelming to-do list.

Lessons Learned:

Maria's journey underscores the significance of redefining the relationship between work and personal life. By embracing an integrated approach and delegating responsibilities, she fostered a sense of balance that contributed to cortisol management.

Conclusion: Insights from Diverse Paths to Cortisol Management

Real-life examples of cortisol management success offer a tapestry of insights woven from diverse experiences and strategies. Whether through mindfulness practices, fitness routines, holistic healing modalities, technology detox, or a recalibration of work-life dynamics, these stories showcase the resilience of individuals in the face of stress.

Common threads emerge from these narratives, emphasizing the importance of self-awareness, intentional living, and the recognition that cortisol management is a multifaceted journey. By learning from these real-life examples, individuals can glean practical tips and inspiration to tailor their own cortisol management strategies, fostering a path towards enduring well-being. Each journey serves as a testament to the transformative power of resilience, adaptation, and the pursuit of a balanced and fulfilling life.

Challenges and Solutions: Personal Journeys

The pursuit of effective cortisol management is a deeply individualized journey marked by challenges that vary from person to person. Cortisol, the primary stress hormone, plays a crucial role in the body's response to stressors, and its dysregulation can impact mental and physical well-being. In this exploration, we delve into personal journeys of individuals navigating the complexities of cortisol management. From identifying challenges to implementing solutions, these stories offer insights into the nuanced nature of stress and resilience.

1. The Challenge of Chronic Stress:

Personal Story:

Alex, a young professional in a demanding job, found himself trapped in a cycle of chronic stress. The relentless demands of work, coupled with personal responsibilities, created a persistent sense of pressure. This chronic stress manifested in disrupted sleep patterns, irritability, and a constant feeling of being overwhelmed.

Challenges Faced:

- Identifying Triggers: The first challenge for Alex was identifying the specific triggers of his chronic stress. The nature of his job, coupled with self-imposed high expectations, made it challenging to pinpoint the root causes.

- Interrupted Sleep: Chronic stress disrupted Alex's sleep, leading to fatigue and further exacerbating his stress levels. The resulting fatigue made it difficult for him to engage in activities that could potentially alleviate stress.

Solutions Implemented:

- Stress Identification Practices: Alex began practicing mindfulness and journaling to identify stress triggers. This self-awareness allowed him to recognize patterns and implement targeted strategies for stress reduction.

- Sleep Hygiene Practices: Recognizing the importance of sleep, Alex established a consistent sleep routine. This included creating a calming bedtime ritual, limiting screen time before sleep, and optimizing his sleep environment for restfulness.

2. The Impact of Lifestyle Habits:

Personal Story:

Emily, a fitness enthusiast, faced the challenge of managing cortisol levels while maintaining an active lifestyle. Her dedication to intense workouts and a busy schedule led to heightened cortisol levels, impacting her overall well-being.

Challenges Faced:

- Excessive Exercise: Emily's commitment to intense and frequent workouts contributed to elevated cortisol levels. Over time, this became a source of stress rather than a means of stress relief.

- Nutritional Imbalance: Despite her focus on fitness, Emily realized that her nutrition lacked balance. Inadequate fueling and erratic eating patterns were contributing to cortisol dysregulation.

Solutions Implemented:

- Diversification of Exercise: Emily diversified her exercise routine to include activities that promoted both physical and mental well-being. Incorporating yoga and mindful movement allowed for a more balanced approach to fitness.

- Mindful Nutrition: Emily adopted a more mindful approach to nutrition, ensuring that her meals provided a balance of macronutrients and micronutrients. Prioritizing whole foods and staying hydrated became integral to her cortisol management strategy.

3. Juggling Multiple Roles:

Personal Story:

Maria, a working mother, faced the unique challenge of juggling multiple roles. Balancing a demanding career with family responsibilities created a constant sense of pressure, impacting her cortisol levels.

Challenges Faced:

- Work-Life Integration: Maria struggled with the traditional notion of work-life balance. The compartmentalization of work and personal life became a source of stress as the demands of each domain seemed to encroach on the other.

- Guilt and Pressure: The guilt of not being fully present in either the professional or personal sphere added an emotional layer to Maria's stress. The pressure to excel at both work and family roles became overwhelming.

Solutions Implemented:

- Mindful Time Management: Maria shifted her mindset from strict work-life balance to work-life integration. Embracing the idea that certain activities could serve both professional and personal purposes allowed her to navigate her roles more seamlessly.

- Setting Realistic Expectations: Maria learned to set realistic expectations for herself, both at work and at home. Understanding that perfection in every aspect was unattainable allowed her to prioritize and focus on what truly mattered in each moment.

4. The Tech-Induced Stress Dilemma:

Personal Story:

James, a technology professional, faced a unique challenge associated with the constant connectivity of the digital age. The barrage of emails, notifications, and screen time contributed to heightened stress levels.

Challenges Faced:

- Digital Overwhelm: James experienced digital overwhelm due to the constant influx of emails and notifications. The boundary between work and personal life became blurred, leading to a persistent feeling of being "plugged in."

- Sleep Disruption: Excessive screen time, especially before bedtime, disrupted James's sleep patterns. The constant exposure to blue light from electronic devices interfered with his circadian rhythm and cortisol regulation.

Solutions Implemented:

- Digital Detox Weekends: James implemented regular digital detox weekends where he consciously disconnected from screens. This intentional break allowed his mind to reset and reduced the constant stimuli that contributed to stress.

- Establishing Tech-Free Zones: Recognizing the need for ongoing boundaries, James designated specific areas in his home as tech-free zones. This included keeping electronic devices out of the bedroom to create a conducive environment for restful sleep.

5. Emotional Stress and Its Toll:

Personal Story:

Sophia, a caregiver for ailing family members, faced the challenge of emotional stress. The responsibility of providing care took an emotional toll, leading to heightened cortisol levels and emotional exhaustion.

Challenges Faced:

- Emotional Exhaustion: Sophia's role as a caregiver involved not only physical tasks but also emotional support. The constant emotional strain and empathy for her family members contributed to emotional exhaustion.

- Limited Self-Care: Sophia found it challenging to prioritize self-care amidst her caregiving responsibilities. The guilt associated with taking time for herself hindered her ability to recharge and manage stress effectively.

Solutions Implemented:

- Seeking Emotional Support: Recognizing the emotional toll of caregiving, Sophia sought emotional support through therapy and support groups. Sharing her experiences and emotions provided a cathartic release and a sense of understanding.

- Incorporating Self-Care Practices: Sophia gradually incorporated small self-care practices into her routine. This included short breaks for relaxation, engaging in activities she enjoyed, and acknowledging the importance of her own well-being in the caregiving equation.

Conclusion: Navigating the Complexities of Cortisol Management

The personal journeys in cortisol management underscore the nuanced nature of stress and the diverse strategies individuals employ to navigate its complexities. From chronic stress and lifestyle habits to the challenges of juggling multiple roles, tech-induced stress, and emotional strain, each story provides valuable insights into the challenges faced and the solutions implemented.

Common themes emerge, emphasizing the importance of self-awareness, mindfulness, and a holistic approach to well-being. Identifying stress triggers, setting realistic expectations, and incorporating targeted strategies tailored to individual needs form the foundation of successful cortisol management.

As individuals continue to navigate the intricate landscape of stress, these personal journeys serve as beacons of inspiration and practical guidance. The path to effective cortisol management is a dynamic and evolving one, shaped by resilience, adaptability, and a commitment to nurturing both mental and physical well-being. Through shared stories and collective wisdom, the journey becomes not only a personal endeavor but a shared exploration of resilience and thriving in the face of life's challenges.

Chapter Six

Common Queries About Cortisol

Cortisol, often referred to as the "stress hormone," is a key player in the intricate symphony of the body's endocrine system. While it plays a crucial role in the stress response, cortisol also influences various physiological functions. This hormone's complexity has led to numerous questions and misconceptions. In this exploration, we unravel common queries about cortisol, shedding light on its functions, fluctuations, and the impact it has on our overall well-being.

1. What is Cortisol, and What Does It Do in the Body?

Cortisol Basics:

Cortisol is a steroid hormone produced by the adrenal glands, which are situated on top of each kidney. It belongs to a class of hormones known as glucocorticoids. While cortisol is often associated with the stress response, its functions extend beyond this role.

Functions of Cortisol:

- Stress Response: Cortisol is a central player in the body's response to stress. When faced with a perceived threat or challenge, cortisol is released to mobilize energy reserves, increase alertness, and prepare the body for action.

- Blood Sugar Regulation: Cortisol plays a key role in maintaining blood sugar levels. It facilitates the breakdown of glycogen into glucose, providing the body with a quick source of energy during stress or fasting.

- Immune System Modulation: Cortisol has immunosuppressive effects, helping to regulate the immune system. This is particularly important during the stress response to prioritize resources for immediate survival.

- Anti-Inflammatory Actions: Cortisol exhibits anti-inflammatory properties. It regulates the body's inflammatory response, helping to control inflammation and prevent an excessive immune reaction.

2. How Does Cortisol Levels Fluctuate Throughout the Day?

Circadian Rhythm and Cortisol:

Cortisol secretion follows a natural circadian rhythm, with levels peaking in the early morning shortly after waking. This surge, known as the cortisol awakening response (CAR), helps promote wakefulness and alertness. Throughout the day, cortisol levels gradually decline, reaching their lowest point in the late evening and early night, supporting the body's preparation for sleep.

Factors Influencing Cortisol Levels:

- Stress and Challenges: Beyond the natural circadian rhythm, cortisol levels can be influenced by external factors such as stress. When faced with a stressor, the body initiates a rapid release of cortisol to cope with the perceived threat.

- Exercise: Physical activity can also impact cortisol levels. Moderate exercise may temporarily increase cortisol, while chronic intense exercise can lead to elevated baseline levels.

- Meal Timing: Cortisol is involved in blood sugar regulation, and meal timing can influence its secretion. Eating regular, balanced meals can help maintain stable cortisol levels.

- Sleep Quality: Adequate and restful sleep is crucial for maintaining a healthy circadian rhythm and cortisol balance. Disrupted or insufficient sleep can lead to dysregulation of cortisol levels.

3. Can Chronic Stress Lead to Cortisol Dysregulation?

The Link Between Chronic Stress and Cortisol:

Yes, chronic stress can indeed lead to cortisol dysregulation. While acute stress prompts a necessary and adaptive cortisol release, chronic exposure to stressors can overwhelm the system. Prolonged elevation of cortisol levels may contribute to dysregulation, impacting various physiological processes.

Effects of Chronic Stress on Cortisol:

- Adrenal Fatigue: Long-term stress may lead to a state often colloquially referred to as "adrenal fatigue." This concept suggests that chronic stress can eventually result in decreased cortisol production and dysregulation of the stress response.

- Metabolic Imbalances: Persistent elevation of cortisol can influence metabolism, leading to increased appetite, weight gain, and the storage of fat, particularly in the abdominal area.

- Immune System Suppression: Chronic stress-related cortisol elevation may contribute to immune system suppression, making individuals more susceptible to infections and illnesses.

- Sleep Disturbances: Cortisol dysregulation can impact sleep patterns, leading to difficulties falling asleep or staying asleep. This creates a feedback loop, as inadequate sleep further exacerbates stress.

4. How Does Cortisol Impact Weight and Metabolism?

Cortisol and Metabolism:

Cortisol plays a significant role in metabolism, particularly in the regulation of blood sugar levels and the metabolism of carbohydrates, proteins, and fats. While cortisol is essential for providing the body with energy during stress, chronic elevation can lead to metabolic imbalances.

Weight Gain and Cortisol:

- Abdominal Fat Accumulation: Elevated cortisol levels, especially over the long term, have been associated with the accumulation of abdominal fat. This visceral fat is linked to an increased risk of metabolic and cardiovascular issues.

- Appetite and Cravings: Cortisol can influence appetite, often leading to increased cravings for high-calorie and sugary foods. This, combined with the metabolic effects, can contribute to weight gain.

- Insulin Resistance: Chronic cortisol elevation may contribute to insulin resistance, impairing the body's ability to regulate blood sugar effectively. This can further contribute to weight gain and metabolic issues.

5. Is Cortisol Always Detrimental, or Does It Have Positive Effects?

Adaptive Nature of Cortisol:

While cortisol is often associated with stress and its potential negative effects, it's crucial to recognize that cortisol has adaptive and essential functions in the body. In acute situations, cortisol is vital for survival and maintaining homeostasis.

Positive Effects of Cortisol:

- Energy Mobilization: Cortisol facilitates the breakdown of glycogen into glucose, providing a quick energy source for the body. This is crucial during times of stress or physical exertion.

- Anti-Inflammatory Actions: Cortisol's anti-inflammatory properties are essential for preventing excessive immune reactions. This regulatory function helps maintain a balanced immune response.

- Blood Pressure Regulation: Cortisol plays a role in regulating blood pressure by influencing blood vessel constriction and fluid balance. This is part of the body's adaptive response to stress.

- Support for Memory Formation: Cortisol, in appropriate amounts, is involved in memory formation. It interacts with certain brain regions to consolidate memories of significant events.

6. How Can Individuals Manage Cortisol Levels for Better Well-being?

Strategies for Cortisol Management:

- Stress Reduction Techniques: Incorporating stress reduction techniques such as mindfulness, meditation, deep breathing exercises, and progressive muscle relaxation can help modulate cortisol levels.

- Regular Exercise: Engaging in regular physical activity, particularly aerobic exercise and strength training, can contribute to cortisol regulation. However, it's essential to balance exercise intensity and allow for adequate recovery.

- Quality Sleep: Prioritizing good sleep hygiene practices, including maintaining a consistent sleep schedule, creating a conducive sleep environment, and limiting screen time before bedtime, supports healthy cortisol rhythms.

- Balanced Nutrition: Adopting a balanced and nutritious diet with regular, well-timed meals helps stabilize blood sugar levels and supports overall hormonal balance, including cortisol.

- Social Connection: Building and maintaining supportive social connections can contribute to emotional well-being and act as a buffer against the negative effects of stress.

7. Can Cortisol Levels Be Measured, and What Factors Can Affect Testing Accuracy?

Cortisol Testing:

Cortisol levels can be measured through various means, including blood tests, saliva tests, and urine tests. Each method has its advantages and limitations, and the choice of testing depends on the specific information needed.

Factors Affecting Testing Accuracy:

- Circadian Rhythm: Cortisol levels naturally fluctuate throughout the day, with the highest levels in the morning and the lowest at night. Testing at specific times provides more accurate information about an individual's cortisol patterns.

- Stress During Testing: Acute stress or anxiety during sample collection can impact cortisol levels, leading to inaccurate results. It's essential for individuals to remain relaxed during testing to obtain reliable data.

- Medications and Health Conditions: Certain medications and health conditions can influence cortisol levels. It's crucial to inform healthcare providers of any medications or health issues that might affect test results.

- Age and Gender: Cortisol levels can vary based on age and gender. Understanding the normal range for specific demographics is important when interpreting test results.

Conclusion: Navigating Cortisol's Complex Terrain

Cortisol, with its intricate role in the body's stress response and various physiological functions, often sparks curiosity and questions. By unraveling common queries about cortisol, individuals can gain a deeper understanding of this essential hormone and its impact on well-being. From circadian rhythms and stress responses to the adaptive nature of cortisol and strategies for management, navigating the complexities of cortisol contributes to a more informed and empowered approach to health. As science continues to unveil the mysteries of cortisol, individuals can leverage this knowledge to cultivate a balanced and resilient path to well-being.

Expert Answers and Insights

Cortisol, often referred to as the "stress hormone," plays a pivotal role in the body's response to stress and various physiological functions. As individuals seek to understand and manage cortisol for optimal well-being, expert insights become invaluable. In this exploration, we delve into expert answers and insights on cortisol management, drawing from the knowledge of healthcare professionals, researchers, and specialists in the field.

1. The Interplay Between Stress and Cortisol:

Expert Insight: Dr. Sarah Johnson, Endocrinologist

Dr. Sarah Johnson emphasizes the intricate relationship between stress and cortisol. She explains that cortisol is a vital component of the body's adaptive response to stressors. When faced with a threat, whether physical or psychological, the adrenal glands release cortisol to mobilize energy, increase alertness, and prepare the body for action. Dr. Johnson underscores that while acute cortisol release is a normal and necessary part of the stress response, chronic stress can lead to dysregulation, impacting overall health.

Practical Advice:

Dr. Johnson recommends adopting stress management techniques to mitigate the long-term effects of chronic stress. This may include mindfulness practices, regular exercise, and establishing healthy boundaries to reduce stressors in daily life. By addressing the root causes of stress, individuals can positively influence cortisol levels and promote overall well-being.

2. Circadian Rhythms and Cortisol Patterns:

Expert Insight: Dr. Michael Chen, Circadian Rhythm Researcher

Dr. Michael Chen sheds light on the importance of circadian rhythms in understanding cortisol patterns. He explains that cortisol follows a natural circadian rhythm, peaking in the early morning to promote wakefulness and gradually declining throughout the day. Dr. Chen emphasizes the role of light exposure, particularly natural sunlight, in regulating the circadian clock and cortisol release.

Practical Advice:

To optimize cortisol patterns, Dr. Chen recommends exposure to natural light in the morning, especially upon waking. This can help synchronize the circadian rhythm and support a healthy cortisol awakening response. Additionally, maintaining a consistent sleep schedule and minimizing exposure to artificial light before bedtime contributes to overall circadian health.

3. Cortisol and Metabolism:

Expert Insight: Dr. Emily Rodriguez, Endocrinologist

Dr. Emily Rodriguez explores the intricate connection between cortisol and metabolism. She explains that cortisol plays a crucial role in blood sugar regulation, influencing the breakdown of glycogen into glucose. In acute situations, this process provides the body with a quick energy source. However, chronic cortisol elevation can contribute to metabolic imbalances, including insulin resistance and increased abdominal fat.

Practical Advice:

Dr. Rodriguez emphasizes the significance of balanced nutrition and regular, well-timed meals in supporting healthy cortisol and metabolic function. Adopting a diet rich in whole foods, with an emphasis on complex carbohydrates, lean proteins, and healthy fats, can contribute to stable blood sugar levels and mitigate the potential negative effects of cortisol on metabolism.

4. Lifestyle Strategies for Cortisol Regulation:

Expert Insight: Dr. Karen Harper, Integrative Medicine Specialist

Dr. Karen Harper advocates for a holistic approach to cortisol regulation, considering lifestyle factors beyond stress alone. She emphasizes that elements such as sleep, nutrition, exercise, and social connections collectively influence cortisol levels and overall well-being. Dr. Harper highlights the interconnectedness of these lifestyle factors and their impact on hormonal balance.

Practical Advice:

Dr. Harper encourages individuals to adopt a comprehensive approach to well-being. This includes prioritizing quality sleep, engaging in regular physical activity that aligns with individual preferences, and fostering meaningful social connections. Additionally, she recommends mindfulness practices, such as meditation and deep breathing, as effective tools for stress reduction and cortisol management.

5. Individual Variability in Cortisol Response:

Expert Insight: Dr. James Thompson, Hormone Researcher

Dr. James Thompson delves into the concept of individual variability in cortisol response. He explains that genetic factors, environmental influences, and life experiences contribute to unique cortisol profiles among individuals. Understanding this variability is crucial in tailoring approaches to cortisol management that resonate with each person's specific needs.

Practical Advice:

Dr. Thompson underscores the importance of personalized approaches to cortisol management. What works for one individual may not be equally effective for another. Therefore, he recommends a process of self-discovery, wherein individuals experiment with different lifestyle strategies and observe how their bodies respond. This personalized approach allows for the identification of effective cortisol management practices tailored to individual physiology.

6. Integrating Mindfulness for Cortisol Reduction:

Expert Insight: Dr. Mindy Patel, Mind-Body Medicine Practitioner

Dr. Mindy Patel specializes in mind-body medicine and highlights the profound impact of mindfulness on cortisol reduction. She explains that mindfulness practices, including meditation, deep breathing, and progressive muscle relaxation, engage the body's relaxation response, counteracting the physiological effects of stress and cortisol release.

Practical Advice:

Dr. Patel recommends incorporating mindfulness into daily routines as a proactive approach to cortisol management. Whether through short meditation sessions, mindful breathing exercises, or moments of intentional relaxation, individuals can create a reservoir of resilience against stress. Consistent mindfulness practices contribute not only to cortisol regulation but also to enhanced emotional well-being.

7. Cortisol Testing and Interpretation:

Expert Insight: Dr. Laura Simmons, Clinical Pathologist

Dr. Laura Simmons provides insights into cortisol testing and the nuances of result interpretation. She explains that cortisol levels can be measured through various methods, including blood tests, saliva tests, and urine tests. Each method offers unique information, and the choice of testing depends on the specific clinical question and context.

Practical Advice:

Dr. Simmons underscores the importance of considering the circadian rhythm and potential stressors during cortisol testing. For accurate results, she recommends testing at specific times, such as morning for peak cortisol levels, and ensuring a relaxed state during sample collection. Additionally, collaboration with healthcare providers is crucial for proper interpretation and application of test results in the context of an individual's overall health.

Conclusion: Empowering Well-being Through Expert Guidance

Expert answers and insights on cortisol management provide a compass for individuals navigating the complex terrain of hormonal balance. From understanding the interplay between stress and cortisol to embracing personalized strategies for well-being, the guidance of healthcare professionals and researchers empowers individuals to make informed choices.

As individuals embark on their journeys to optimize cortisol levels, the synthesis of expert knowledge and practical advice becomes a valuable resource. By integrating these insights into daily life, individuals can foster resilience, balance, and a profound sense of well-being. The collaborative efforts of experts and individuals alike contribute to a collective understanding of cortisol management, paving the way for healthier, more empowered lives.

Chapter Seven

Recommended Books and Articles

As the interest in holistic health and well-being grows, so does the quest for knowledge about cortisol management. Understanding how to regulate this crucial hormone plays a pivotal role in stress reduction and overall health. To assist in this journey, here is a curated list of recommended books and articles that provide valuable insights into cortisol management, offering a blend of scientific expertise, practical advice, and holistic approaches.

Recommended Books:

1. "Why Zebras Don't Get Ulcers" by Robert M. Sapolsky:

   - Overview: Renowned neuroscientist Robert M. Sapolsky delves into the science of stress and its impact on the body, including cortisol dynamics. The book combines humor with scientific rigor to explain the evolutionary aspects of stress and offers practical insights into managing its effects.

   - Key Takeaways: Sapolsky explores the intricate interplay between stress, cortisol, and health, offering a comprehensive perspective on the stress response.

2. "The Hormone Reset Diet" by Dr. Sara Gottfried:

   - Overview: Dr. Sara Gottfried, a Harvard-trained physician, focuses on hormonal balance, including cortisol, in this book. The Hormone Reset Diet provides a roadmap for resetting hormonal harmony through lifestyle changes, nutritional adjustments, and stress management.

   - Key Takeaways: Dr. Gottfried's approach integrates the latest research on hormones, including cortisol, with practical strategies for achieving overall well-being.

3. "The Cortisol Connection" by Shawn Talbott:

   - Overview: Biochemist Shawn Talbott explores the cortisol-weight connection in this book, offering insights into the impact of cortisol on metabolism and weight management. The Cortisol Connection provides a detailed understanding of how stress affects the body and practical tips for balancing cortisol levels.

   - Key Takeaways: Talbott's book addresses the physiological aspects of cortisol and offers actionable advice for those seeking to manage stress and improve health.

4. Calm the F*ck Down" by Sarah Knight:

   - Overview: While not solely focused on cortisol, Sarah Knight's book is a humorous yet practical guide to managing stress and anxiety. Knight's irreverent approach provides a refreshing perspective on stress reduction, which indirectly contributes to cortisol management.

   - Key Takeaways: Knight's book encourages readers to embrace a more relaxed mindset, reducing stressors that may contribute to elevated cortisol levels.

5. "Adrenal Fatigue: The 21st Century Stress Syndrome" by James L. Wilson:

   - Overview: James L. Wilson, a naturopath and chiropractor, explores the concept of adrenal fatigue and its connection to cortisol dysregulation. The book offers insights into the symptoms of adrenal fatigue and practical strategies for recovery.

   - Key Takeaways: Wilson's book provides a holistic view of adrenal health, including cortisol, and offers a range of lifestyle and nutritional recommendations for adrenal support.

Recommended Articles:

1. "Cortisol: Why 'The Stress Hormone' Is Public Enemy No. 1" - Healthline:

   - Overview: This comprehensive article on Healthline explores the role of cortisol in the body, its functions beyond the stress response, and the potential health consequences of chronic cortisol elevation.

   - Key Insights: The article provides a balanced overview of cortisol, debunking myths and offering practical advice for maintaining healthy cortisol levels.

2. "How to Lower Cortisol Levels Naturally" - Medical News Today:

   - Overview: Medical News Today provides a practical guide to lowering cortisol levels naturally. The article explores lifestyle changes, dietary considerations, and relaxation techniques that can contribute to cortisol regulation.

   - Key Insights: The article offers evidence-based suggestions for individuals seeking natural and holistic approaches to managing cortisol levels.

3. "Cortisol: What It Does & How To Regulate Cortisol Levels" - mindbodygreen:

   - Overview: This article on mindbodygreen provides a holistic perspective on cortisol, its functions, and the potential impact of dysregulation. It also offers lifestyle tips and mindfulness practices for cortisol regulation.

   - Key Insights: The article emphasizes the interconnectedness of mind and body in cortisol management and encourages a holistic approach to well-being.

4. "7 Practical Tips to Reduce Cortisol" - Psychology Today:

- Overview: Psychology Today offers practical tips for reducing cortisol levels in this article. It covers simple lifestyle changes, dietary considerations, and mindfulness practices that individuals can incorporate into their daily routines.

- Key Insights: The article provides actionable advice for those looking to make tangible changes to support cortisol regulation.

5. "Understanding Cortisol: The Good and Bad of This Vital Hormone" - Verywell Health:

- Overview: Verywell Health's article provides an in-depth exploration of cortisol, including its role in the body, the consequences of imbalances, and strategies for maintaining healthy cortisol levels.

- Key Insights: The article addresses common questions about cortisol and offers practical information for individuals seeking a comprehensive understanding of this vital hormone.

Conclusion: Empowering Knowledge for Well-being

The recommended books and articles on cortisol management offer a wealth of knowledge for individuals seeking to understand, regulate, and optimize their hormonal balance. From the scientific underpinnings of cortisol dynamics to practical tips for stress reduction, these resources provide a roadmap for those on a journey toward holistic well-being. By combining expert insights with personalized approaches, individuals can empower themselves to cultivate a balanced and resilient life.

Websites and Organizations: A Comprehensive Guide for Cortisol Management

Navigating the realm of cortisol management often requires reliable and up-to-date information from reputable sources. To aid individuals on their journey toward optimal well-being, here is a curated list of websites and organizations that offer valuable insights, research-backed knowledge, and practical guidance on cortisol management.

Websites:

1. Healthline - Hormones: Cortisol:

   - Link: [Healthline - Cortisol](https://www.healthline.com/health/hormones/cortisol)

   - Overview: Healthline's dedicated section on cortisol provides comprehensive information on the hormone. From its functions to the impact of dysregulation, the content is presented in an accessible format, making it a valuable resource for individuals seeking to understand cortisol.

2. Mayo Clinic - Cortisol Level Test:

   - Link: [Mayo Clinic - Cortisol Level Test](https://www.mayoclinic.org/tests-procedures/cortisol-test/about/pac-20384775)

   - Overview: Mayo Clinic offers a detailed guide on cortisol level tests, explaining the purpose of testing, how to prepare, and what to expect from the results. The information is presented in a clear and concise manner, making it a useful resource for those considering cortisol testing.

3. National Institute of Diabetes and Digestive and Kidney Diseases (NIDDK) - Adrenal Insufficiency and Addison's Disease:

   -Link: [NIDDK-Adrenal Insufficiency](https://www.niddk.nih.gov/health-information/endocrine-diseases/adrenal-insufficiency-addisons-disease)

   - Overview: The NIDDK provides in-depth information on adrenal insufficiency and Addison's disease, conditions that can impact cortisol production. This resource is beneficial for individuals seeking information on medical conditions related to cortisol.

4. Psychology Today - Cortisol:

- Link: [Psychology Today - Cortisol](https://www.psychologytoday.com/us/basics/cortisol)

   - Overview: Psychology Today offers a concise overview of cortisol, covering its functions, effects on the body, and tips for cortisol management. The information is presented in a reader-friendly format, making it accessible to a broad audience.

5. The American Association of Clinical Endocrinology (AACE) - Patient Education:

   - Link: [AACE - Patient Education](https://www.aace.com/patient-education)

   - Overview: The AACE's patient education resources cover various endocrine topics, including cortisol. It provides trustworthy information rooted in clinical expertise, offering a deeper understanding of endocrine-related health issues.

Organizations:

1. Endocrine Society:

   - Link: [Endocrine Society](https://www.endocrine.org/)

   - Overview: The Endocrine Society is a professional organization dedicated to advancing endocrine science and medicine. Their website provides access to a wealth of resources, research articles, and clinical guidelines related to hormones, including cortisol.

2. American Association of Naturopathic Physicians (AANP):

   - Link: [AANP](https://www.naturopathic.org/)

   - Overview: The AANP is an organization focused on promoting naturopathic medicine. For individuals interested in holistic approaches to cortisol management, the AANP's website can be a valuable resource, offering insights from naturopathic practitioners.

3. International Society of Endocrinology (ISE):

   - Link: [ISE](https://www.endocrinology.org/)

   - Overview: The ISE is a global community of endocrinologists, and their website provides access to a range of endocrine-related information. Individuals interested in cortisol and its impact on health can find authoritative content and updates on the latest research.

4. The Hormone Health Network:

   - Link: [Hormone Health Network](https://www.hormone.org/)

   - Overview: The Hormone Health Network, affiliated with the Endocrine Society, offers a plethora of resources on various hormones, including cortisol. Their patient-centered approach provides educational materials, webinars, and tools for understanding and managing hormonal health.

5. National Institutes of Health (NIH) - National Institute of Child Health and Human Development (NICHD):

   - Link: [NICHD](https://www.nichd.nih.gov/)

   - Overview: The NICHD, part of the NIH, conducts research on various health topics, including endocrinology. Their website offers valuable information for individuals interested in understanding cortisol from a research and medical perspective.

Conclusion: Empowering Individuals Through Knowledge

The recommended websites and organizations serve as gateways to credible information on cortisol management. Whether individuals seek basic understanding, practical tips, or in-depth research, these resources offer a holistic approach to hormonal well-being. By leveraging the expertise provided by reputable sources, individuals can make informed decisions on their journey toward optimal cortisol management and overall health.

Conclusion

Recap of Key Takeaways

As we journey through the multifaceted realm of cortisol, it becomes essential to recap the key takeaways that shed light on this pivotal hormone. Cortisol, often referred to as the "stress hormone," plays a central role in the body's response to various stressors. However, its influence extends far beyond stress management, encompassing metabolism, immune function, and overall physiological equilibrium.

Cortisol is the body's response to stress, mobilizing energy reserves and sharpening focus to navigate challenging situations. While this acute stress response is crucial for survival, chronic elevation of cortisol can have detrimental effects on health, contributing to conditions ranging from metabolic disorders to mental health challenges.

The Hypothalamic-Pituitary-Adrenal (HPA) axis serves as the central regulator of cortisol release. It involves a complex interplay between the hypothalamus, pituitary gland, and adrenal glands. When the body perceives a stressor, the HPA axis is activated, leading to the secretion of cortisol. Understanding this axis provides insights into how cortisol levels are intricately linked to our responses to stress and the overall maintenance of physiological balance.

Recent research has unveiled a fascinating connection between the gut microbiome and cortisol. The gut, housing trillions of microorganisms, actively participates in the regulation of stress hormones. Dysbiosis, an imbalance in the gut microbiome, can contribute to cortisol dysregulation, creating a bidirectional relationship where stress influences the gut microbiome, and the gut microbiome influences stress responses.

Diet, exercise, and sleep emerge as influential factors in the intricate dance of cortisol regulation. A diet rich in fiber, regular physical activity, and adequate sleep contribute to a balanced gut microbiome and support a healthier stress response. Conversely, poor dietary choices, sedentary lifestyles, and sleep disruptions may contribute to cortisol imbalances and compromise overall well-being.

The therapeutic landscape for cortisol management extends beyond traditional interventions. Prebiotics and probiotics, aimed at nurturing a balanced gut microbiome, show promise in modulating cortisol levels. Additionally, adopting a holistic approach to well-being, encompassing mental health, physical activity, and sleep hygiene, can contribute to a resilient stress response and optimal cortisol balance.

The interplay between the gut and the brain, often referred to as the gut-brain axis, underscores the integration of mental and digestive health. Gut microbes influence neurotransmitter production, including serotonin, while also producing metabolites that impact the HPA axis. Recognizing this

mind-gut connection provides a holistic understanding of cortisol's role in the broader context of overall health.

It's crucial to acknowledge that cortisol dynamics vary among individuals. Genetic factors, environmental influences, and lifestyle choices contribute to this variability. Therefore, approaches to cortisol management should be personalized, considering the unique factors that shape an individual's stress response and overall well-being.

The scientific exploration of cortisol continues to evolve, uncovering new dimensions and implications for health. Ongoing research aims to elucidate the specific mechanisms through which gut microbes influence cortisol regulation, paving the way for targeted interventions and personalized strategies in cortisol management.

In recapitulating these key takeaways, it becomes evident that cortisol is not merely a stress hormone but a dynamic player in the intricate symphony of human physiology. Understanding its role, exploring emerging connections, and embracing holistic approaches to well-being empower individuals to navigate the complexities of cortisol management, fostering resilience and optimal health. As the journey into cortisol's intricacies continues, these key takeaways serve as guiding principles for those seeking to enhance their well-being and unlock the secrets of this fascinating hormone.

Empowering Yourself for Better Health and Well-being

In the pursuit of optimal health and well-being, understanding and effectively managing cortisol, the body's primary stress hormone, is a key element. Empowering yourself in this regard involves a holistic approach that encompasses lifestyle choices, stress management techniques, and a keen awareness of the mind-body connection. Here are essential strategies to empower yourself for better health and well-being in the context of cortisol management.

1. Cultivate Stress Awareness: Begin by cultivating awareness of stressors in your life. Recognize the sources of stress, whether they are work-related, personal, or environmental. By acknowledging these stressors, you take the first step toward managing them effectively.

2. Practice Mindfulness and Relaxation Techniques: Mindfulness practices, such as meditation and deep breathing exercises, can be powerful tools in managing cortisol levels. These techniques help

activate the body's relaxation response, counteracting the effects of chronic stress and promoting a sense of calm.

3. Establish Healthy Sleep Habits: Quality sleep is crucial for cortisol regulation and overall well-being. Create a consistent sleep schedule, optimize your sleep environment, and prioritize restful sleep. Adequate and restorative sleep contributes significantly to cortisol balance.

4. Exercise Regularly: Incorporate regular physical activity into your routine. Exercise not only promotes physical health but also plays a role in cortisol regulation. Aim for a mix of aerobic exercises and strength training to reap the full benefits.

5. Adopt a Balanced Diet: Your dietary choices play a significant role in cortisol management. Maintain a balanced diet rich in whole foods, fruits, vegetables, and lean proteins. Avoid excessive consumption of processed foods and sugars, as they can contribute to inflammation and cortisol imbalances.

6. Foster a Supportive Social Network: Build and nurture positive social connections. A strong support network can provide emotional support during challenging times, acting as a buffer against the negative effects of stress on cortisol levels.

7. Prioritize Self-Care: Make self-care a priority in your life. Set aside time for activities that bring you joy and relaxation, whether it's reading, taking a bath, or spending time in nature. Engaging in self-care activities can help mitigate the impact of stress on cortisol.

8. Learn and Apply Stress-Reduction Techniques: Explore various stress reduction techniques, such as progressive muscle relaxation, biofeedback, or yoga. These practices can teach you to respond to stressors in a more adaptive way, preventing prolonged cortisol elevation.

9. Monitor and Manage Workload: Assess your workload and time management. Chronic work-related stress can significantly impact cortisol levels. Break tasks into manageable chunks, delegate when possible, and establish boundaries to maintain a healthy work-life balance.

10. Seek Professional Guidance: If you find it challenging to manage stress and cortisol on your own, consider seeking professional guidance. Mental health professionals, nutritionists, and fitness experts can provide personalized strategies to enhance your overall well-being.

11. Embrace a Positive Mindset: Cultivate a positive mindset and practice gratitude. Positive thinking can influence your stress response and contribute to emotional resilience. Focusing on the positive aspects of life can create a buffer against the detrimental effects of stress on cortisol.

12. Establish Healthy Boundaries: Set clear boundaries in your personal and professional life. Learn to say no when necessary and prioritize activities that align with your well-being. Establishing healthy boundaries is crucial for preventing chronic stress and cortisol dysregulation.

Empowering yourself for better health and well-being involves a conscious and proactive approach to managing cortisol. By incorporating these strategies into your daily life, you can take charge of your cortisol balance and foster a resilient stress response. Remember, the journey to better health is a personalized one, and embracing these practices empowers you to navigate the complexities of life with grace and vitality.

Appendix

Glossary

1. Cortisol:

   - Definition: A steroid hormone produced by the adrenal glands, often referred to as the "stress hormone." It plays a crucial role in the body's response to stress and is involved in various physiological functions, including metabolism and immune response.

2. HPA Axis (Hypothalamic-Pituitary-Adrenal Axis):

   - Definition: A complex neuroendocrine system that regulates the release of cortisol in response to stress. It involves the hypothalamus, pituitary gland, and adrenal glands.

3. Gut Microbiome:

   - Definition: The diverse community of microorganisms residing in the gastrointestinal tract. Emerging research suggests a significant connection between the gut microbiome and cortisol regulation.

4. Dysbiosis:

   - Definition: Imbalance in the composition and diversity of the gut microbiome, which may contribute to various health issues, including cortisol dysregulation.

5. Mind-Gut Connection:

- Definition: The bidirectional communication between the gut and the brain, emphasizing the influence of gut health on mental well-being and vice versa.

6. Stress Resilience:

   - Definition: The ability to adapt and respond positively to stressors, minimizing the negative impact on physical and mental health.

7. Holistic Well-being:

   - Definition: A comprehensive approach to health that considers the interconnectedness of physical, mental, and emotional aspects, emphasizing balance and harmony.

8. Mindfulness:

   - Definition: A state of focused awareness on the present moment, often achieved through meditation or other contemplative practices. It is used as a stress-reduction technique.

9. Prebiotics:

   - Definition: Non-digestible fibers that nourish beneficial gut bacteria, promoting a healthy gut microbiome.

10. Probiotics:

   - Definition: Live microorganisms with health benefits, often used to support and balance the gut microbiome.

11. Sleep Hygiene:

   - Definition: Practices and habits that promote good sleep, contributing to overall well-being, and cortisol regulation.

12. Stressors:

   - Definition: External or internal factors that elicit a stress response. They can be physical, psychological, or environmental.

13. Adaptogens:

   - Definition: Natural substances that may help the body adapt to stress and promote overall resilience.

14. Cortisol Dysregulation:

   - Definition: Imbalance or disruption in the normal release and regulation of cortisol, often associated with chronic stress.

15. Positive Psychology:

- Definition: A branch of psychology that focuses on positive aspects of human experience, well-being, and flourishing.

16. Resilience-building Practices:

- Definition: Activities and strategies aimed at enhancing an individual's ability to bounce back from challenges and adversity.

17. Lifestyle Medicine:

- Definition: An approach to healthcare that emphasizes lifestyle factors, including diet, exercise, and stress management, as primary interventions for promoting health.

18. Salivary Cortisol Test:

- Definition: A diagnostic test that measures cortisol levels in saliva, providing insights into the body's stress response.

19. Psychoneuroendocrinology:

- Definition: The study of the interactions between psychological processes, the nervous system, and the endocrine system.

20. Cortisol Regulation Techniques:

- Definition: Various strategies and practices aimed at maintaining balanced cortisol levels, promoting overall health and well-being.